ThinStead

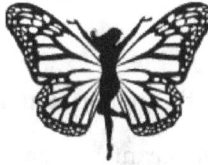

The ultimate plan to finally lose the weight, feel great, and quit dieting forever

By KATHLEEN LAMMENS, C.H.T.

Printed in the United States of America

Cover design by Steve Sharon

The names and details of some individuals have been changed.

FIRST EDITION

ISBN 978-0-615-64968-9

10 9 8 7 6 5 4 3 2 1

For everyone who has struggled with losing the same twenty pounds over and over again. This is for you.

Contents

Contents

Acknowledgements

ThinStead could not have been published without the assistance and encouragement of many wonderful people to whom I am tremendously grateful.

First and foremost, I'd like to thank my incredible family. My parents, Barbara and Art, have been a constant source of love, support and strength in my life. Laurie and Joe, your bountiful creative talents and quick wit continuously serve as an inspiration to me. I love you all more than words can say.

I also offer my deep appreciation to my many amazing friends for their friendship, generosity, and encouragement. They each nourish my soul, nurture my dreams, and bring a sense of adventure to my life.

I would also like to extend my sincerest appreciation to Rob Hall for lending his keen editorial eye, invaluable wisdom and general muse-ness.

My heartfelt thanks belong to Steve Sharon for his graphic arts genius and talent for bringing the vision of the book to life.

A debt of gratitude is also owed to the pioneers who worked painstakingly to bring the emotional freedom techniques to the world, as well as the many spiritual teachers I've met and whose works I've read along the way. They have all contributed greatly to the healing of the world.

Finally, I am deeply grateful to all my clients who so graciously shared their stories and experiences, so that readers could also achieve miracles in their own lives. Thank you!

Introduction

The ThinStead Program for Permanent Weight Loss

Welcome! Thank you for purchasing the ThinStead program for permanent weight loss. ThinStead is a mind/body, therapy-based weight loss program designed to eliminate food addiction and compulsive eating easily and rapidly, allowing you to experience permanent weight loss. It's designed to help you finally achieve freedom from the nightmarish cycle of food addiction, compulsive eating and weight gain. It's been my experience working with clients that as they address the emotional causes that drive their compulsive eating behavior, they begin to experience life in a more peaceful and joyful way. Many often find a passion for life that they never had before. I invite you, too, to experience a more joyful, passionate life starting here, starting right now!

I struggled with weight gain for over 20 years myself. I tried low calorie diets, low carb diets, the HCG diet - you name it. It seemed like I gained and lost the same extra weight many times over. After my last diet, I had lost 50 lbs and I felt great. But all of those good feelings were tied to how much weight I'd lost. It wasn't long after I stopped dieting that I began to pile the weight back on – very rapidly. At a rate of about 5 -10 pounds a month. I realized then that no diet was ever going to fix the REASON I was overweight – my compulsive eating behavior. There had to be another solution, and I was determined to find it.

The exercise gurus like to tell us that the reason we're overweight is because we eat too much. They say it's a simple equation of too much food and too little exercise. And that's partially true. But they don't acknowledge the real reason we eat too much in the first place. We eat to stuff our feelings and we eat to ease the pain and anxiety hidden deep within. We eat to fill the gaping hole inside of us. We eat to keep from having to feel the feelings that we think will crush us if we were to acknowledge them. Compulsive eating is born of fear, deep sadness, anxiety, deprivation and lack of love.

In my own weight loss struggle, I found that when I finally addressed these underlying emotions in my own life, the compulsive eating went away on its own - without struggle, or strife or deprivation of any kind. That realization led me to develop the ThinStead program. ThinStead is different from diets. Diets really don't work. After all, how many diets have you undertaken in your life? Was the weight loss permanent, or did you find yourself packing the pounds back on again as soon as you stopped? The diet industry is a multi-billion dollar industry for a reason. That's because there are a lot of repeat customers!

There's also an alarming trend toward the acceptance and marketing of weight loss surgery these days. Any kind of surgery always carries a risk, and while it may be a lifesaver for the morbidly obese, often it's not the miracle cure it's touted as being. Post-surgical complications range from relatively mild, like the inability to metabolize certain nutrients and fiber, hair loss, gastric dumping and acid reflux, to the more dangerous such as anemia, chronic pain, internal hernias, blood clots, bowel obstructions, intussusception and even death. In many cases, the stomach just stretches back to its original size over time. I know several people who have had the surgery done and it will affect how they live for the rest of their lives. In fact, a relative of a dear friend of mine passed away from a drug dependency brought on by the extreme chronic pain she experienced after her weight loss surgery.

I firmly believe that bariatric surgery is not worth the inherent dangers. The benefits do not, in my opinion, outweigh the risks. For example, on my very last diet I lost weight at a rate of .6 pounds a day. There was some intermittent cheating involved, but I did manage to lose 50 pounds in a little over 3 months. It was a very hard core diet, to be sure. But the results that dieters obtain are on par with those obtained from weight loss surgery. On the Mayo Clinic's website they state:

"Within the first two years of surgery, you can expect to lose 50 to 60 percent of your excess weight."

Let's do a little math. It is generally accepted that a person qualifies for bariatric surgery if they have 100 pounds of excess weight for a man or 80 pounds for a woman. So let's assume you are female with 80 pounds to lose and have a best case scenario outcome (60% loss) according to Mayo. That means you would have lost 48 lbs within the first two years after surgery. And yet, with diet alone, I was capable of losing 50 in under 4 months. I just don't see where the rate of weight loss offered by bariatric surgery justifies the risk of possible death. The whole bariatric surgery industry is predicated upon the erroneous assumption that people have *no control* over their eating behavior and must be forcibly starved into submission.

The Mayo website goes on to say:

"Gastric bypass surgery can be an effective treatment for obesity, and most people do lose weight after the procedure. But you'll always be at risk of regaining the weight you do lose, even years later. To help reach your weight-loss goal and prevent weight regain, it's crucial to make lifestyle changes along with having gastric bypass surgery."

Basically they're saying that bariatric surgery is not a magic bullet or a miracle cure. At some point we'll need to stop putting too much of the wrong kind of foods into our bodies and adopt a healthier lifestyle. So why not go ahead and make the lifestyle changes up front, the easy way, and skip the dangerous surgery altogether? ThinStead will show you how!

ThinStead and EFT: The Permanent Solution

ThinStead is a program designed to permanently eliminate compulsive eating behavior. ThinStead utilizes a step by step plan to address each of the emotional issues contributing to your own personal food addiction problem. Using your own introspection, combined with specially designed written exercises and a particular Energy Psychology therapeutic modality called EFT (Emotional Freedom Techniques) or "Tapping", you will be able to quickly eliminate the emotional drivers which cause your out of control eating behavior – once and for all.

The ThinStead Process

You + EFT + ThinStead Exercises =

Freedom from Food Addiction

One of my clients, Karen, says of her experience with ThinStead:

"When I started tapping on my childhood experiences of never being able to have what I wanted, and never feeling like I was listened to, things really started coming up. One night I had a dream about a tiny white pony that was starving. I was running around frantically trying to get people to give me food and water for this little pony. When I woke up in the morning I was sobbing for this pony. I had no idea why it affected me so much. But I couldn't stop crying, so I decided to just go with it. I tapped on 'the suffering of the pony' and then 'the suffering of all the animals' and the tears just kept coming. Now I realize that the pony represented me. But I just kept tapping until the tears finally stopped."

"At that moment, a peace came over me. It was like a cloud had lifted. The world literally became clearer and fresher. I remember going out to the grocery store later in the day, and all the people seemed to be looking at me and smiling. It was like they were seeing me for the first time. It was a totally spiritual experience. From that moment on, my compulsive eating stopped. I used to crave chocolate and other sweets all the time. But I don't any more. I've lost 12 pounds so far without even really trying. ThinStead is amazing!"

Karen's experience shows the importance that our dreams can sometimes have in our healing journey. They represent our deepest, innermost emotions. Because of their symbolic nature, we can tap on themes that emerge from our dreams and address the emotions contained within them. We can even tap on emotions that we're having in the moment, without even really knowing where they are coming from, like when we're in the middle of a food craving.

When I asked Karen about what her life was like after she finished the ThinStead program she had this to say: "I'm in control of my eating now. I don't feel guilty or ashamed after I eat and being around food doesn't cause me anxiety. Food is no longer the enemy. I feel completely free!"

In this book, you'll find instructions on the pressure point tapping protocol, lists of emotional aspects for tapping, and daily exercises that will help you rapidly work through the emotions which are causing your overeating. If you faithfully follow the exercises in this book, I guarantee you will see results. But remember, you'll only get out of the program as much as you put into it. So for the best possible results, make sure you're fully committed to losing your food addiction before you start reading this book. In my practice, my weight loss clients are typically able to work through their issues in anywhere from 1 to 3 sessions. Watching my clients be released from their compulsive overeating and go on to lead happy, peaceful and transformed lives has been the most fulfilling part of my career. It is my fondest hope that the ThinStead program will do the same for you.

So get ready to begin your own journey to permanent weight loss, inner peace and tranquility. It all starts now!

Chapter 1

How ThinStead Works

Over the years, I've found many useful therapeutic tools. One of the most miraculous is Energy Psychology. Energy Psychology is a mind/body healing modality that combines emotional, talk-based therapy with gentle tapping on certain acupressure points on our body. I know the idea of Energy Psychology may be a new concept to some people at first, but the results I've witnessed in my work have been rapid and astounding.

What Energy Psychology can do that cognitive behavioral therapy or psychotherapy can't, is actually **remove** the emotional pain and trauma that we carry within our bodies. Traditional talk therapy is useful to help you identify *why* you're sad or frightened or angry, but it does nothing to remove those feelings. Visualization and hypnosis are also helpful, but it's difficult to install positive beliefs without first removing the negative.

A few minutes after trying Energy Psychology, you will be utterly convinced. Negative, uncomfortable emotions simply evaporate into thin air. Using the ThinStead program has allowed me to eliminate my own compulsive eating behavior, increase my passion and zest for living, and experience weight loss for life. I know it can do the same for you.

There are several modalities within the Energy Psychology field, but one of the fastest acting and most elegant is EFT, or Emotional Freedom Techniques. I've seen EFT resolve problems in a session or two that might take many years to resolve in traditional psychotherapy. EFT, developed by Stanford engineer Gary Craig, happens to be one of the easiest Energy Psychology modalities to learn. It's a system whereby you tap gently with your fingertips on several acupressure points on your body, as you call to mind uncomfortable feelings or memories, while you say brief anchoring phrases.

The pressure points that we use in EFT are linked to some of the same major energy meridians that acupuncturists have been using since the second century BC. As you gently tap on these acupressure points, the negative emotions that you're holding within your body are released from your energy system for good. Some people have deep physical relaxation responses as they feel these emotions disappear forever. For example, yawning happens to be one of my own responses to emotional release. It's also not uncommon to experience cleansing tears as well while tapping away negative emotions.

The reason that EFT works so quickly is that if you address the correct feeling or belief (which are called "aspects") underlying a given emotional or physical problem, the problem itself will "collapse" and all symptoms will dissipate. This is great news! Instead of just addressing the symptom of overweight, we can go directly to the cause of our food addictions – our deepest emotions.

Fortunately, the emotional drivers underlying compulsive eating behavior are fairly consistent and predictable from person to person and frequently center around the emotions of grief, sadness, anxiety, anger, deprivation, lack of love and low self-esteem. In developing the ThinStead program, I compiled hundreds of the most typical emotional "aspects" held by compulsive overeaters, while letting the healing power of EFT stand on its own. This comprehensive list of emotional components, combined with your own introspection, gives you a systematic tool for addressing the emotions which may be contributing to your own compulsive eating behavior. Once you have released these deep-seated emotions, your once compulsive eating behavior will be a thing of the past!

Scientific Research

Though there has been ample anecdotal evidence surrounding the effectiveness of Energy Psychology since the 1970's, it wasn't until more recently that the scientific evidence to back it up began to emerge. Scientific research is very often funded by pharmaceutical companies or academic institutions, neither of which have a particularly vested interest in proving the efficacy of a holistic healing modality. Also, it is inherently difficult to scientifically measure emotions, and we are mostly left to rely on self-report by study participants. However, in a research paper published in 2004, Joaquin Andrade, M.D. and David Feinstein, Ph.D. reported their comprehensive findings resulting from experiments conducted in Energy Psychology (tapping).

In a series of experiments involving over 29,000 patients in South America receiving treatment for anxiety and other emotional disorders, it was determined that tapping methods of treatment received results that were equal to or superior to conventional means of treatment – either Cognitive Behavioral Therapy (CBT) or medication. Not only that, but results were achieved faster by patients in the experimental group who received the tapping treatment than by those receiving conventional treatment. Furthermore, the tappers were substantially less likely to relapse by a follow-up at one year, than those receiving standard treatment.

These findings were further supported by EEG brain scans. Dr. Andrade and his team scanned the brains of participants, analyzing the ratio of brain wave frequencies (alpha, beta, and theta) before, during and after treatment for Generalized Anxiety Disorder. They found that while the patients receiving CBT and Energy Psychology therapy both showed an improvement toward normal brain wave function, it took more therapy sessions to achieve results with CBT than with tapping (average of 15 sessions for CBT, versus 3 sessions for tapping). Moreover, at a one year follow-up, the patients receiving the tapping treatment were more likely to have maintained normal brain wave ratios, as compared to the patients receiving CBT.

In addition, Dr. Andrade found that patients receiving anti-anxiety medications as their primary treatment did not exhibit the same noticeable beneficial changes in their brain wave patterns as did the tapping patients, even when they had a reduction in symptoms from the drugs. These results suggest that the anti-anxiety medication was *suppressing the symptoms* of anxiety without actually addressing the underlying brain imbalances. It is clear from Dr. Andrade's research that **Energy Psychology is an extremely powerful tool for dealing with emotional issues** from the standpoint of speed, effectiveness and permanence. The success of EFT in dealing with negative emotions makes it a perfect tool for overcoming addictive, emotionally driven eating behaviors!

While the precise mechanism behind Energy Psychology's amazing success has yet to be fully identified, there are several hypotheses that have been put forth. Acupuncture, which is a

5,000 year old discipline still widely practiced today, is based on the idea that the human body is surrounded by, and generates its own energy field. This energy field is capable of being measured by scientists with devices called Squid Magnetometers, or superconducting quantum interference devices. Modern medical diagnostic tools such as MRIs, EKGs and EEGs are even designed around this concept of measuring differences in the human electromagnetic field.

Experiments conducted using the radioisotope Technetium-99 injected into acupuncture points have even been able to map these meridians (Kovacs FM, et al. Experimental study on radioactive pathways of hypodermically injected technetium-99m: Journal of Nuclear Medicine 1992; 33:403-407.). I would encourage anyone who is interested in reading more about recent research into acupuncture to check out http://www.ncbi.nlm.nih.gov/pubmed/. It has a wonderful database of published studies.

In Traditional Chinese Medicine, it is generally accepted that each of the body's major energy meridians, or channels, is associated with specific emotional themes (for example, the liver channel is often associated with the emotion of anger). It has been suggested by proponents of acupuncture that tapping on the energy meridians, while focused on a specific emotional problem, may restore the energy balance in the disrupted energy meridian responsible for modulating that particular emotion.

Tapping on acupuncture points can also be examined from a strictly biological perspective as well. Brain imaging techniques have been able to identify signals emanating from structures within the limbic system, such as the amygdala and hippocampus, when a person experiences a negative emotion. Some research scientists postulate that the afferent signals produced by tapping

11

on acupuncture points intercept the signals produced by the brain and cause a shift in the biochemical foundations underpinning a particular emotion.

One of the distinct advantages that tapping has over traditional talk therapy is its ability to transmit sensory signals directly to the amygdala, the brain structure associated with generating the body's fight or flight response and storing fearful emotional memories. There are many chemicals and hormones involved in the regulation of the fear response in the amygdala. One of the major players is gamma-aminobutyric acid, or GABA. GABA is the chief inhibitory neurotransmitter in the human central nervous system, and is responsible for suppressing the excitation response of neurons in the amygdala. According to Joseph LeDoux Ph.D., sometimes the suppressive ability of GABA may become compromised, resulting in panic and anxiety disorders.

The pharmaceutical industry has developed many drugs to try and combat this problem. Valium and other benzodiazepines were developed to increase the efficiency of GABA. SSRI antidepressants were created in order to boost serotonin, a neurotransmitter that excites the cells that produce GABA. Drugs like Prozac work by increasing the amount of serotonin available at brain synapses. Interestingly, studies at the Martino Center for Biomedical Imaging have shown that acupuncture increases serotonin levels, as well as reducing levels of norepinephrine and dopamine, two biological markers associated with stress and pain.

The bottom line is that Energy Psychology has a strong scientific basis for its efficacy. And EFT is the most exciting healing modality I have encountered to date. It has literally helped millions of people worldwide. I chose to incorporate EFT into the ThinStead program in order to help food addicts like myself gain rapid, permanent relief from their compulsive eating behavior. Thinstead has been my miracle, and I know it can be yours too. So if you are fully committed to ending the continuous cycle of yo-yo dieting once and for all, let's begin!

Chapter 2

Personal Food Addiction Assessment

The ThinStead process is a profound spiritual and emotional journey which leads you back to yourself. It's a journey back to emotional health, sanity and peace. And like any significant spiritual journey, in order to chart where we're going, it's helpful to look at where we've been and how we got to where we are now.

To help you prepare for the work ahead, I've created the following self-assessments and questions that are designed to help you identify your current feelings surrounding your life, food, and eating behaviors. Taking time to read through them and answer them thoroughly and completely will give you a clear idea of how much your compulsive eating is truly affecting your life. It may make you a little sad at first to see how much of an impact your food addiction really has on your happiness and quality of life. Don't worry. That's actually a great thing, because getting in touch with these emotions will give you an excellent place to start when you begin to tap on your emotional eating triggers. By the end of this program, the unhappy memories which may now elicit so much pain will no longer have the same negative charge for you. So, if you're ready to take the first step in your journey, read on.

Please complete the following assessment relating to your eating behaviors. Take as much time as you need to answer each question fully.

Emotions and Eating Behavior

	Never	Rarely	Sometimes	Frequently	Always
I am aware of my own needs and emotions.					
I work through my emotions without turning to food.					
I eat frequently throughout the day.					
I crave specific foods to feel good.					
I binge eat at least once a day.					
I am obsessed about what I will eat for future meals.					
I eat when I'm hungry and stop when I'm full.					
I make healthy, nutritious food choices.					
I am physically active.					
I feel anxious every day.					
I feel safe and secure in the world.					
I feel a sense of purpose in my life.					
I love and accept myself.					

Please read the following questions and rate your current life satisfaction level:

Life Satisfaction

	Not at all 1	Not very 2	Somewhat 3	Very 4	Extremely 5
How happy are you with your career/job?					
Are you satisfied with your current financial state?					
How happy are you with the state of your physical health?					
How happy are you with your romantic life?					
How happy are you with your emotional life?					
How happy are you with your family relationships?					
Do you feel spiritually fulfilled?					
Do you feel creatively fulfilled?					
Are you satisfied with the amount of fun and enjoyment in your life?					
Do you feel like you are contributing to society at large?					
Do you have a set of defined goals for your life?					
How happy would you say you are with your life overall?					

After filling out each assessment, how do you feel about your quality of life in general? Had you realized just how much of an impact your food addiction had on your life? Have you gone to any extreme measures to hide your food addiction from others?

Jot down some of your thoughts here:

_____

_____

_____

_____

The following questions are designed to get you thinking about your childhood and what other conditions, situations and incidents may have contributed to your current food addiction problem. Take as much time as you need to answer each question. Feel free to use a pad of paper if you need more room to list your thoughts. In fact, the more detailed your answers are, the easier it will be later to tap on the personal issues and triggers which are the root of your food addiction.

How long have you had a weight problem?

_____

_____

_____

When did you first recognize it had become a problem?

_____

_____

_____

_____

Is there anything of significance that you can recall which started you on the path to overeating?

_____

_____

_____

_____

How old were you when you first started overeating? What was happening in your life when you began having a weight problem?

_____

_____

_____

_____

Can you think of some other situations or events that may have contributed to your weight problem?

_____

_____

_____

If there was an emotional cause behind your overeating, what would it be? If you don't know, just take a wild guess.

_____

_____

_____

_____

If your food addiction had a message for you, what would it be?

_____

_____

_____

_____

_____

Do others in your family struggle with weight? If so, who?

_____

_____

_____

_____

What would you change about your childhood if you could?

_____

_____

_____

_____

Was there any physical, emotional or sexual abuse in your childhood? If so, how have you dealt with it up until now?

_____

_____

_____

_____

When you have an urge to binge, what foods are your "go to" or comfort foods? List as many as you can think of.

_____

_____

_____

_____

Congratulations! You've just taken the first step in your healing journey. You deserve a great deal of credit for your courage and motivation to finally conquer your food addiction. By following the ThinStead program, you're actually performing a profound act of self care. You are saying to yourself, "I matter." From this moment on, you'll be eliminating your anxiety, guilt, shame and sadness, and creating more peace, happiness and self-esteem.

In the next chapter you'll learn more about the tool you'll be using to overcome your food addiction once and for all.

Chapter 3

EFT – The Miracle Tool

Now that you've done the preliminary work of examining how food addiction and compulsive eating have affected your life up to this point, it's time to learn about the tool you'll be using to remove the emotional causes of your addiction. EFT is a healing modality that's been around in one form or another for over 25 years, and it's very easy to learn. Gary Craig designed it to be very "user friendly". It's not even necessary for you to believe in EFT in order for it to work.

To eliminate the emotional causes of our overeating, we will be tapping gently with our fingertips on acupressure points on our hand, head and torso. These points coincide with several energy meridians used in traditional acupuncture. The principle behind EFT is the same as in acupuncture; that is, a disruption in the flow of our body's energy system can result in negative emotions, as well as physical ailments. In the same way acupuncture has been used successfully for thousands of years to manipulate the human energy field, we'll be using gentle acupressure to release the negative emotions that we hold in our bodies.

When we tap, we will use the tips of the first two fingers of our dominant hand – the index and middle finger. We use two fingers in order to increase the surface area that we'll be able to tap on. Now let's take a look at the acupressure points we'll be using.

The Acupressure Points

The first acupuncture point we will tap on is on the outside of your hand, on the pinky side. It's on the percussion, where you would connect with something if you were going to give it a karate chop. Consequently, we refer to it as the karate chop point, or **KC**, for short. Typically we tap with the first two fingers of our dominant hand on the KC point of the opposite hand.

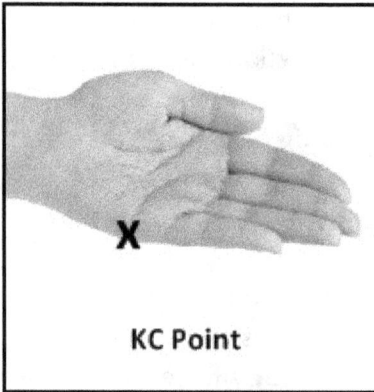

KC Point

The next tapping point is called the eyebrow point, or **EB**, for short. It is located where the bridge of your nose meets the inside edge of your eyebrow.

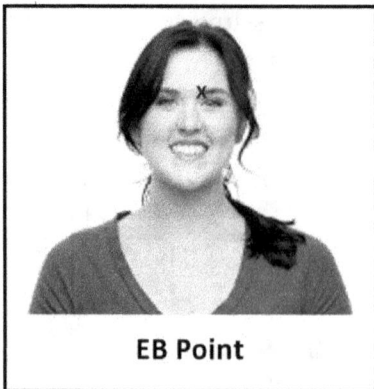

EB Point

Next is the point on the side of the eye, or **SE** point, and it is located along the orbit bone about level with your pupil.

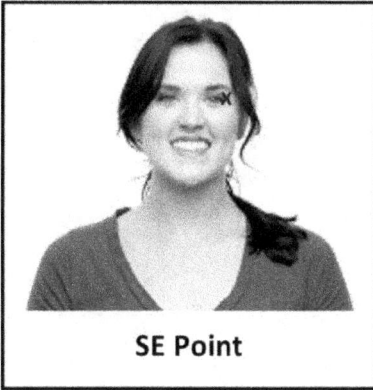

SE Point

Next is the under eye point, or **UE**, which is also along the orbit bone, directly beneath your pupil.

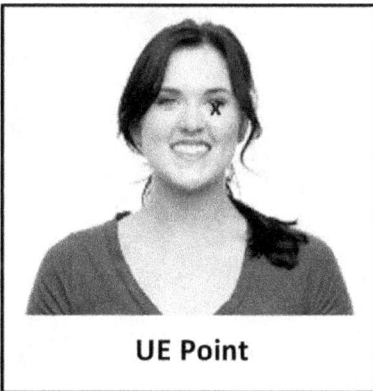

UE Point

Next there's the point under your nose, or **UN**, in the middle, exactly halfway between your nostrils and upper lip.

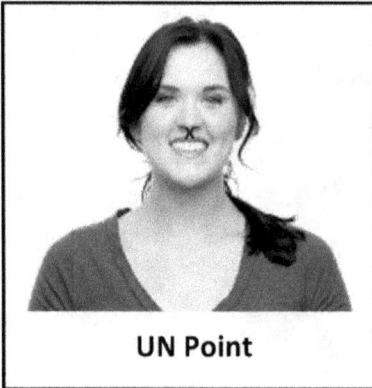

UN Point

After that is the chin point, or **CH**, which is located in the indentation between your lower lip and point of your chin.

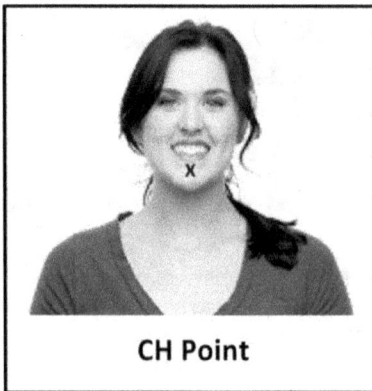

CH Point

Next is the collar bone point, or **CB**, for short. To find it, place your fingers in the u-shaped notch below your throat (about where you would tie a necktie). Now move your fingers down 1 inch and over 1 inch. This is where the CB point is located. As you can see, it's not exactly located on your collar bone, but the name is descriptive enough to give you the gist. It's technically located where the sternum and first rib meet.

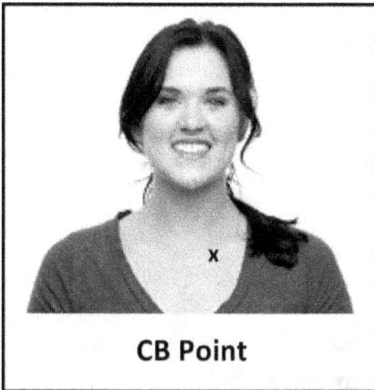

CB Point

After that is the underarm point, or **UA**. It's located on the side of your body, about 4 inches or so below your armpit, at the same level as your nipple for men, or in the middle of your bra strap for the ladies.

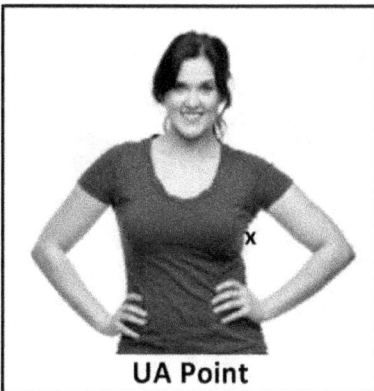

UA Point

And finally there's the point directly in the center of the top of your head (**TH**).

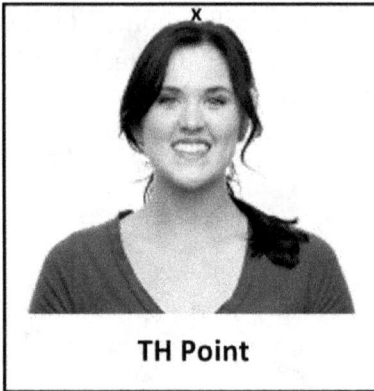

TH Point

Now that you're familiar with the points we'll be using, do a quick run through by tapping on each point 5-7 times with two fingers, in the order you learned them.

KC   Karate Chop Point
EB   Eyebrow
SE   Side of Eye
UE   Under Eye
UN   Under Nose
CH   Chin
CB   Collar Bone
UA   Under Arm
TH   Top of Head

Do it a couple of times, until it begins to feel like second nature. It's important to remember to be gentle, because we'll be doing a lot of tapping and you don't want to make yourself sore. Also keep in mind that you can tap on either side of your body, so if you feel like switching sides at any time, that's fine. Generally we'll tap 5 to 7 times on each spot, but don't get hung up on the numbers or counting. Just spend a little time on each spot to make sure you cover it. EFT is a very forgiving modality and it will work even if you don't get it perfectly right.

The Basic Recipe Explained

Now that you have the tapping points down, it's time to review the basic three part procedure we will be using throughout the book. It is referred to as the EFT "Basic Recipe".

Rate Your Intensity

The first step in the EFT process is to give our problem an intensity rating on a scale of 1 to 10. For example, let's say it's the middle of the afternoon and you are having an intense craving for your favorite snack food. It's quite probable that you're experiencing a high level of intensity, perhaps even a level 10 on the intensity scale. Assess your level of intensity.

0 = No emotional intensity or craving at all
5 = Moderate intensity or craving
10 = Maximum intensity – the most you have ever felt

Our goal, using tapping, is to eventually reduce the level of intensity to a zero. Rating the issue before you tap lets you know how much tapping you have to do to achieve relief. Assess your intensity after each full round of tapping to decide if you've released the issue, or if you need to do another round or two.

The Set Up

The second part of the formula is called the "Set Up Phrase". The set up phrase identifies the current problem, emotion, or memory you're tapping on. For example, let's say your favorite afternoon snack food is a candy bar and you're experiencing a powerful craving. We begin by tapping our karate chop point while **repeating the set up phrase 3 times** like this:

KC   Even though I have this powerful craving for a candy bar, I deeply and completely love and accept myself.

KC   Even though I have this powerful craving for a candy bar, I deeply and completely love and accept myself.

KC   Even though I have this powerful craving for a candy bar, I deeply and completely love and accept myself.

The set up phrase serves 3 functions. First, it helps us to focus our attention on the problem at hand. Second, it helps us affirm that even though we have this problem, we still accept ourselves just as we are. And third, the set up phrase is useful for undoing what we call "psychological reversal". Usually if we are experiencing an area of life where we are stuck, there is a fair amount of psychological resistance surrounding the subject, and in Energy Psychology we are said to be "reversed". The set up phrase is designed to neutralize any mental and energetic resistance we have toward releasing the problem.

The easiest way to perform the set up is to simply repeat the same set up phrase 3 times. However it's also possible to vary the wording of the set up phrase a little to prevent boredom, as long as the core meaning of the 3 phrases remains essentially the same. You'll notice I've done that with the set up phrases throughout the book. Also, when saying your set up phrases, really put emotion into it. Really try to elicit the feeling of loving and accepting yourself. It makes your tapping even more effective.

Sometimes we may feel some resistance to the phrase "I deeply and completely love and accept myself." We may not feel like we love ourselves. We may not even be able to conceive of loving and accepting ourselves. If that's the case we can begin by using some other phrases that we don't have as much resistance to. If we simply let ourselves be "willing" to learn how to love ourselves, that's enough to allow change to start to happen. If you feel a strong resistance to saying that you love and accept yourself, try some of the set up phrases below to start with:

Even though I have this problem...

I am willing to learn to love and accept myself.

I am willing to begin to love and accept myself.

I am willing to be open to the possibility of loving and accepting myself.

I am willing to remember that God loves me and accepts me just as I am.

These alternate set up phrases can help move you in the right direction. After saying them for a while, you will feel much more comfortable about actually loving and accepting yourself and will be able to use the original phrasing.

The Tapping Rounds

The third part of the basic recipe is called the tapping "Rounds". This is where we tap on the 8 points on our torso and head while repeating the reminder phrases. The reminder phrases are any words that you say to keep yourself tuned into the problem you're tapping for. They can consist of anywhere from 1 to 10 words or more. They can be just a few words or entire phrases. The reminder phrases should be directly related to the problem at hand. You can either repeat the same reminder phrase at each tapping point, or you can use multiple reminder phrases to tune in to different aspects of the issue being tapped on. At times throughout the book we'll be alternating between positive and negative statements while doing the tapping rounds. This will allow us to focus on and release negative emotions, while simultaneously instilling positive affirmations.

The goal of the tapping rounds is to continue tapping on the 8 acupressure points until the emotional charge or discomfort surrounding the issue is reduced to a level zero. This is why you should check in after every round of tapping and assess your current level of intensity to see if you've reduced it down to, or near, zero.

NOTE: I've included a one page EFT Quick Guide on the following page which recaps the process. Please feel free to tear it out and carry it with you to have as a handy reference.

EFT Quick Guide

Identify the issue you want to work on. **RATE** your level of intensity from 0-10.

SET UP — Repeat 3 X while tapping on KC Point

"Even though I have this issue, I deeply and completely love and accept myself."

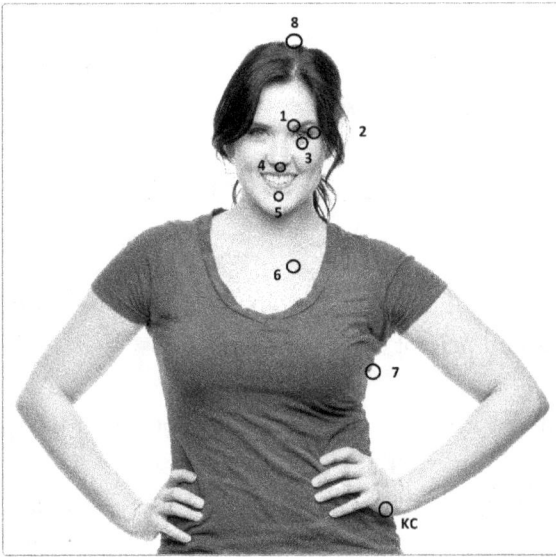

TAPPING ROUNDS
(Tap 5 to 7 times on each point)

1. Eyebrow
2. Side of Eye
3. Under Eye
4. Under Nose
5. Chin
6. Collar Bone
7. Under Arm
8. Top of Head

Three Step Process In Brief

So to recap, this is the **3 Step Process** we will be using:

1. **Assess your level of intensity** on the subject at hand on a scale from 1 to 10.

2. **Repeat the set up phrase 3 times** while tapping on your Karate Chop point:

KC   Even though _____, I deeply and completely love and accept myself.

KC   Even though _____, I deeply and completely love and accept myself.

KC   Even though _____, I deeply and completely love and accept myself.

3. Do as many **rounds of tapping** as you need to bring your intensity down, while repeating the reminder phrases, on the following points. Remember to tap 5-7 times on each.

    EB   Eyebrow
    SE   Side of Eye
    UE   Under Eye
    UN   Under Nose
    CH   Chin
    CB   Collar Bone
    UA   Under Arm
    TH   Top of Head

Here's an example of how the whole process works:

Say you're watching television, and you see an advertisement for a major pizza chain. Now you can't get the idea of a piping hot, cheesy pizza out of your head. You develop a major craving and you want to eliminate it. Here's how you do that.

First, identify how much you want that pizza. How strong is your craving? Is it a 10? An 8?

Next begin tapping on your KC point while performing the set up phrase, 3 times:

KC   Even though I have this craving for pizza, I deeply and completely love and accept myself.

KC   Even though I can't get the idea of pizza out of my head, I deeply and completely love and accept myself.

KC   Even though I have this tremendous urge for pizza, I deeply and completely love and accept myself.

Now tap on the tapping points using the reminder phrases. Tap on each point 5-7 times.

EB	Eyebrow Point	this pizza craving
SE	Side of Eye Point	this overwhelming urge for pizza
UE	Under Eye Point	this need for pizza
UN	Under Nose Point	this craving for hot pizza
CH	Chin Point	this pizza craving
CB	Collar Bone Point	this cheesy, gooey pizza craving
UA	Under Arm Point	this urge for pizza
TH	Top of Head Point	this strong craving for pizza

Initially, do 2 or 3 rounds of this tapping. Now stop and assess your current level of craving. Did it drop? Is it more like a 3 or 4? Is it even lower? Tap another couple of rounds with the following set up and reminder phrases:

KC   Even though I have this *remaining* craving for pizza, I deeply and completely love and accept myself.

KC   Even though I have this *remaining* pizza craving, I deeply and completely love and accept myself.

KC   Even though I have this *remaining* craving for hot pizza, I deeply and completely love and accept myself.

EB	Eyebrow Point	this remaining craving
SE	Side of Eye Point	this remaining craving
UE	Under Eye Point	this remaining craving
UN	Under Nose Point	this remaining craving
CH	Chin Point	this remaining craving
CB	Collar Bone Point	this remaining craving
UA	Under Arm Point	this remaining craving
TH	Top of Head Point	this remaining craving

When we get our level of intensity down fairly low, we often use the word "remaining" to get at the last little bit of emotion we may be harboring surrounding the subject.

Remember as you do the tapping rounds, you should try to get your level of craving as low as you can. Ideally to a zero. Your goal regarding the pizza is to feel like you can "take it or leave it". The more specific you can make your set up AND reminder phrases, the better. So really get into it! Think about your favorite qualities of that pizza, describe why you like it out loud.

Embellishing with your own personal touches can be really helpful in reducing emotional intensity even further. Your own tapping round might look something like this:

Set Up

KC   Even though I crave this hot, cheesy, mushroom and pepperoni pizza, I deeply and completely love and accept myself.

KC   Even though I need a hot, cheesy, mushroom and pepperoni pizza, I deeply and completely love and accept myself.

KC   Even though I really want a hot, cheesy, mushroom and pepperoni pizza, I deeply and completely love and accept myself.

Tapping Rounds

Possible Reminder Phrases:

EB	Eyebrow Point	This craving
SE	Side of Eye Point	This pizza
UE	Under Eye Point	This cheesy pizza
UN	Under Nose Point	Warm, doughy pizza
CH	Chin Point	Chewy, soft crust
CB	Collar Bone Point	Saucy, cheesy pizza
UA	Under Arm Point	Delicious pizza
TH	Top of Head Point	Comforting Pizza

The idea is to touch on all the reasons why you are craving this particular food. Remember, the reminder phrases don't always have to be the same during one tapping round. They can be varied and alternated for each tapping point, according to your feelings regarding the topic you're tapping on. Remember to tap on each point about 5–7 times. Tap until your intensity is reduced to zero.

It's important to realize that sometimes we can't get to zero on a particular topic right away. But as we continue to tap on other, related aspects, we can eventually get to a level zero and reach a place of peace on a given issue.

A Few Words About Effective Tapping

For the set-up, you'll be using some variation of the following phrases. At first it may not be easy to say the words out loud. Initially, it may feel like you're lying. If that's the case, you may choose to omit the word "love" for now. But as you repeatedly say these phrases, they'll begin to feel more true for you. As time goes on, you will be able to add the word love back into the set-up phrase.

Here are some of the most common set up phrases:

Even though _____, I deeply and completely accept myself.

Even though _____, I deeply and completely love and accept myself.

Even though _____, I deeply and profoundly love and accept myself.

Even if _____, I choose to completely love and accept myself anyway.

It's also acceptable to switch the order of the phrase on occasion just to keep from getting bored, like so:

I choose to love and accept myself anyway, even if _____.

It's very important that you **always** include the **accepting** portion of the phrase when you're tapping on the set up phrase, in order to release the negative emotions associated with the subject you're tapping on.

NOTE: A little later in the book, I'll begin **short handing** the set up phrases for your ease of reading, like so:

Even though I eat when I'm bored

Even though I eat when I'm anxious

However, you should still **complete the set up phrase** with the ending "I deeply and completely love and accept myself" <u>every</u> time you are tapping on a set up phrase. Tapping on our acceptance of ourselves is crucial to our healing process.

Helpful Hints

I've found that doing EFT with another person, such as a therapist, can be very helpful. That's because often the other person can give insights and point out things that aren't readily apparent to us. But there are some things we can do to get these same benefits while tapping on our own.

Always Remember To Be Specific

One of the most important things to keep in mind is that every emotional blockage we carry has many aspects to it. And the more specific we can be in our set up and reminder phrases the better. For example, let's say you remember a time when you were a child that your father spanked you and scolded you for something that you weren't aware was wrong at the time. You're likely to have some negative feelings about that experience. You might be sad, or disappointed or angry about your father yelling at or hitting you. You would also have experienced various sensations of sight, or sound, smell or even touch. Each one of these thoughts, emotions and sensations is an "aspect" of the experience.

So for the above example, we might use set up phrases similar to these:

Even though my father scolded me for going outside, I deeply and completely love and accept myself.

Even though my father whacked me on my butt and it really hurt, I deeply and completely love and accept myself.

Even though I didn't know why my father hit me, I deeply and completely love and accept myself.

Even though I can't believe he hit me, I deeply and completely love and accept myself.

Even though he was really loud and angry, I deeply and profoundly love and accept myself.

Even though he said I was bad, and sent me to my room without dinner, I deeply and completely love and accept myself anyway.

To get even more specific, you could also tap on his facial expressions, your own physical sensations, or any other details which stood out in your mind at the time of the event. The point is to break each topic, memory or event down into smaller chunks – each of which is an aspect contributing to the overall hurt. Being very specific becomes increasingly important the more traumatic an event is. Anyone who has experienced childhood trauma or abuse should be especially conscious about tapping on the details surrounding an abusive event. This will serve to release the hurt much more rapidly.

Shifting Aspects

Please also keep in mind that as you work through an issue or traumatic event, **your emotions surrounding the issue at hand are likely to shift.** The way to deal with this is after a few rounds of tapping on an issue, take a moment to stop and notice your remaining feelings regarding the subject. Let's say you're tapping for some emotional event from your childhood that you're feeling sad about. Perhaps after you do a couple rounds of tapping, you no longer feel sad. But you might now feel a little angry or resentful about having had to go through that experience. You would then do a few rounds of tapping for the new emotion of anger, until you released it as well.

Personalize The Process

Throughout the book, I'll lead you through a series of tapping which follows a strategic plan and addresses specific sets of underlying emotional aspects relating to food addiction. You will also be asked to answer questions that are designed to help you get at the root of your own compulsive eating behavior. The program is designed to have a smooth, logical flow created to root out the main causes of food addiction and compulsive/binge eating. However, they are by no means the totality of all the aspects that could be contributing to your own overeating problem. That's why it's very important for you to do thorough introspection and answer each question as fully as you can.

Frequently while we're tapping, other thoughts, memories, emotions and insights will come up. So, if at any time while tapping you receive an insight that is not listed in the suggested tapping phrases provided, please feel free to momentarily stop, and *tap on the information you received in your insight*. Your insights are likely to be highly specific, personal and relevant to your own food addiction. These insights are links in the chain of healing. If the new insights are coming too fast for you to remember them all, feel free to stop and jot them down on a piece of paper.

In addition, it is very important to *frame your set up and reminder phrases to reflect your own thoughts and wording*. For example, if the phrase provided is, "Even though I'm so fat", but in your head you constantly say to yourself, "I'm such a tub of lard," a better phrase for you would be; "Even though I'm such a tub of lard, I deeply and completely love and accept myself." The goal is to make our set up and reminder phrases as personal as we can to match our own experience. As food addicts, we are frequently brutally unkind in what we think and say about ourselves and our bodies. Using these very same unkind words in our tapping work will help clear out the underlying aspects more effectively and rapidly.

Checking In

The way you'll know if you are done with an issue is if you no longer feel an emotional charge surrounding it. That's why after you've tapped on all the aspects you can think of for a given topic, you should check in and determine your level of emotional intensity on a scale of 1 – 10. We're shooting for a zero here. So maybe you've tapped on an issue that caused you great sadness. You started out at a 10 on the scale, but you've managed to bring yourself down to a 2. You no longer really feel sad about it, but perhaps now you realize that you have a little lingering anger for having had to go through the experience. You would then tap again for that anger and bring yourself down to a zero. Remember to check, check and check again. It's the only way to know if you've really released an issue.

Proper Preparation

Because we're working directly with the body's energy system, it's important that we be well hydrated when we're performing EFT. Our bodies are electromagnetic in nature, so make sure and get your 8-10 eight ounce glasses of clean water every day. It's also very important to remove cell phones from our work space, and move away from other electronics or appliances that generate an electro-magnetic field (like computers with wi-fi, or wireless routers) when we're doing tapping work.

Be Gentle

The ThinStead program is all about being kind and gentle with yourself. Examining your feelings and re-experiencing old emotional wounds is very hard work. It's important to be patient with yourself, your emotions, and the process as it unfolds. I recommend working your way through the book at a relaxed pace. Each section will deal with some very heavy emotions. It's worthwhile to take your time and process what you've learned from each exercise, as well as examine any new emotions that crop up. A chapter per day is probably sufficient, as each chapter deals with different facets of your addiction.

One of the nice things about using EFT to deal with emotional issues is that we can also tap for our **fear** of dealing with certain issues in advance of actually working with them directly. If you've had an especially traumatic childhood, you may be feeling some trepidation or discomfort about dealing with those difficult issues. If that's the case, then I would encourage you to tap on your fear of finally dealing with your past.

You might begin with a set up phrase like "Even though I'm afraid to deal with my abuse" or "Even though I'm scared to look at my past" or "Even though I don't want to relive the molestation, I deeply and completely love and accept myself." Then do a few rounds of tapping for "this fear" or "this anxiety", until you bring your anxiety about dealing with the issue to as close to zero and you can get. This will clear the way to allow you to really deal honestly with the issue and get at its core aspects.

So if you're ready, let's begin the journey to peace and freedom together!

Chapter 4

Tapping on the Problem

Before we begin tapping on the various aspects of our food addiction, we should first do some energetic "house cleaning". While the simplified EFT basic recipe is extremely effective for the majority of my clients straight out of the gate, I have encountered a few people who were experiencing extreme psychological reversal surrounding their weight issues. I find it is therefore worthwhile to deal with this problem at the outset. Even if we're not massively psychologically reversed surrounding the issue of food addiction, it doesn't hurt to have an added insurance policy.

People with predominantly negative thought patterns or people who suffer from addictions are frequently psychologically "reversed". Psychological reversal is a polarity reversal which disrupts the body's energy system that is caused by negative thinking patterns. These energy disruptions can interfere with and impede the EFT tapping process. So I usually recommend doing a meridian balancing technique as a precautionary measure before beginning to work on food addiction problems, other types of addictions, or emotional traumas. Here's a technique to quickly neutralize extreme psychological reversal.

Tapping For Extreme Psychological Reversal

The following technique is called the Collar Bone Breathing Exercise and it was developed by Dr. Callahan in order to correct any energy reversals that may exist within the body. In order to do it, you'll need to know one additional acupressure point. In EFT it is called the gamut point. It is located on the back of both hands, and is a half inch behind the midpoint between the knuckles at the base of your ring finger and pinky.

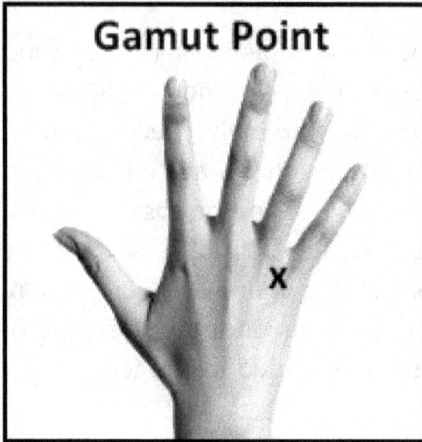

Gamut Point

Before doing this exercise, sit down and get comfortable, away from any electronic devices in your house, and make sure you are adequately hydrated with water.

During this exercise you'll tap on your gamut point while inhaling and exhaling in a specific way. As you inhale through your nose and exhale through your mouth, you'll breathe in and out in increments. As you do the exercise, make sure to hold your arms out to your sides, away from body. Your arms shouldn't rest against your body. Also, you want your fingertips and knuckles to be the only things making contact with your body. If you're ready, let's begin:

Collar Bone Breathing Exercise

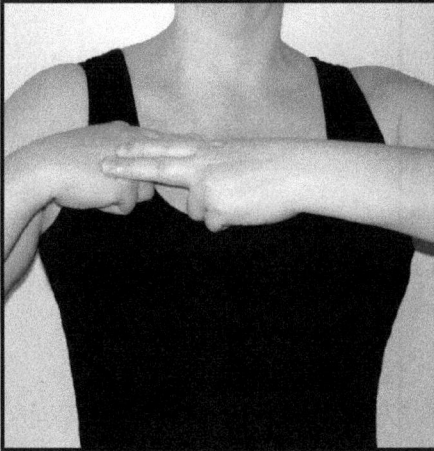

1.   Place the tips of your right index and middle finger on your right collar bone point. (Remember you are holding your arms out to the side so they do not rest on your body.) With your left index and middle finger, continuously tap the gamut point on your right hand while doing the following breathing exercise:

Breathe half way in and hold for 7 taps
Breathe all the way in and hold for 7 taps
Breathe half way out and hold for 7 taps
Breathe all the way out and hold for 7 taps
Breathe normally for 7 taps

2. Place the tips of your right index and middle finger on
    your left collar bone point. With your left index and
    middle finger, continuously tap the gamut point on your
    right hand while doing the same breathing exercise as
    before:

    Breathe half way in and hold for 7 taps
    Breathe all the way in and hold for 7 taps
    Breathe half way out and hold for 7 taps
    Breathe all the way out and hold for 7 taps
    Breathe normally for 7 taps

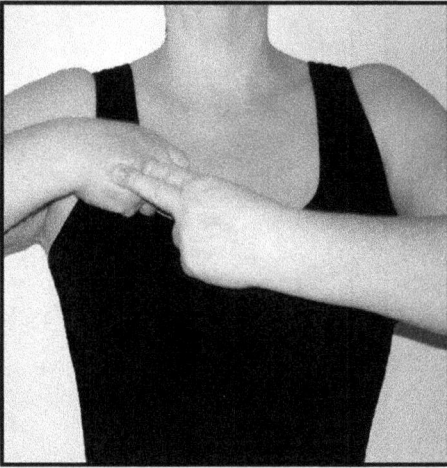

3.   Now bend the fingers on your right hand so that the second joint or knuckles are prominent, and place the index and middle finger knuckle points on your right collar bone point, and tap on the gamut point with your left hand while breathing like so:

Breathe half way in and hold for 7 taps
Breathe all the way in and hold for 7 taps
Breathe half way out and hold for 7 taps
Breathe all the way out and hold for 7 taps
Breathe normally for 7 taps

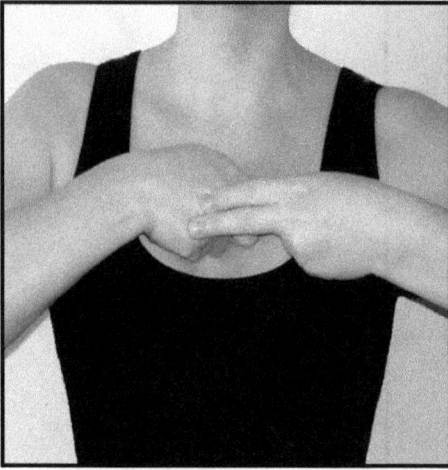

4.   Place those same knuckles on your left collar bone point and continue tapping the gamut point on your right hand while breathing as follows:

Breathe half way in and hold for 7 taps
Breathe all the way in and hold for 7 taps
Breathe half way out and hold for 7 taps
Breathe all the way out and hold for 7 taps
Breathe normally for 7 taps

You've just completed half the circuit. Now do the same 4 steps using your opposite hands to tap your gamut point and press your collar bone point:

1. Place the tips of your left index and middle finger on your right collar bone point. (Remember you are holding your arms out to the side so they do not rest on your body.) With your right index and middle finger, continuously tap the gamut point on your left hand while doing the breathing exercise:

    Breathe half way in and hold for 7 taps
    Breathe all the way in and hold for 7 taps
    Breathe half way out and hold for 7 taps
    Breathe all the way out and hold for 7 taps
    Breathe normally for 7 taps

2. Place the tips of your left index and middle finger on your left collar bone point. With your right index and middle finger, continuously tap the gamut point on your left hand while doing the breathing exercise above.

3. Now bend the fingers on your left hand so that the second joint or knuckles are prominent, and place the index and middle finger knuckle points on your right collar bone point, and tap on the gamut point with your right hand while doing the breathing exercise above.

4. Place those same knuckles on your left collar bone point and continue tapping the gamut point on your left hand while doing the breathing exercise.

Now you are done clearing up any severe energetic reversals and you're ready to begin the process of eliminating your food addiction once and for all. The collar bone breathing technique can be used any time you feel like you're not making any further progress on a particular issue because you may be psychologically reversed on it. Don't worry, the collar bone breathing exercise can't make you become "reversed", so there's never any harm in doing it if you feel you want to, and it's always very relaxing.

Tapping For Food Addiction In General

Now we'll begin to unravel the roots of your food addiction by tapping in a systematic way, beginning with general issues relating to food addiction and then progressing to more specific emotional aspects. The first aspect we'll begin tapping on is the general problem of food addiction itself. It's very likely that you have some strong emotions about having a food addiction and being overweight. Hitting the problem head on will make it easier to tap on more specific aspects later, as wells as break down some of the barriers you might have to your recovery.

At this point, some people who are students of the Law of Attraction might be curious as to why we tap and focus on negative thoughts and emotions while doing EFT. The answer is that the Universe is very intelligent. It knows what your deepest emotions are at any given moment. So, if you're busy repeating positive affirmations, but you're subconsciously vibrating the emotions of grief, fear, anger or lack, the Universe will know it. It can't be outsmarted. The beauty of EFT is that it acts as a bridge to positive emotions. We can't deny our true feelings, and by using EFT we can release all of our stored negative emotions, once and for all. Our new emotional freedom then allows us to move into the space of positive vibration, where we can more easily attract what we truly want into our lives.

First we'll start with some basic tapping designed to reduce your resistance to getting over your problem. Remember to follow the formula you learned in Chapter 3; assess the intensity of your emotions surrounding the issue, repeat the set up phrases 3 times, perform tapping rounds with reminder phrases (2 or 3 rounds minimum) until intensity is reduced to zero.

On a scale of 1 to 10, how intense are your emotions surrounding overcoming your weight problem? Do you doubt your ability to conquer your food addiction? Do you feel skeptical about whether tapping will work for you? While EFT does work whether one believes in it or not, harboring lingering doubts can sabotage your progress by keeping you from becoming fully engaged in your healing process. Your doubts make you less able to access the emotions and insights which need to be explored in order to release your food addiction.

Let's begin by tapping along with the following set up phrases:

SET UP

While tapping on the KC Point:

KC   Even though I don't believe tapping will help, I'm willing to deeply and completely love and accept myself.

KC   Even though I don't believe I can tap away my food addiction problem, I deeply and completely love and accept myself anyway.

KC   Even though I'm not convinced tapping will work, I choose to deeply and completely love and accept myself anyway.

TAPPING ROUNDS

Now do 2 to 3 rounds of tapping on the 8 points:

EB	Eyebrow	I'm not sure EFT will work
SE	Side of Eye	I'm not sure it will work for me
UE	Under Eye	I'm not sure I can tap away my problems
UN	Under Nose	My obsession with food is very strong
CH	Chin	But I choose to believe I can be healed
CB	Collar Bone	I choose to believe I can release my fears
UA	Under Arm	I want to release my anger and sadness
TH	Top of Head	I choose to believe I can release my food addiction for good

Continue tapping on the following set ups and reminder phrases. Remember to always complete the set up phrases with the words "deeply and completely love and accept myself" or some variation which communicates your self-acceptance. Try and do a minimum of 2 to 3 rounds of tapping for each of the set ups provided, and tap on each point 5-7 times.

SET UP

While tapping on the KC Point:

KC Even though I don't believe I can get over my food addiction, I'm willing to deeply and completely love and accept myself.

KC Even though I don't believe I can get over my weight problem, I deeply and completely love and accept myself anyway.

KC Even though I don't think it's possible for me to be a thin person, I choose to deeply and completely love and accept myself anyway.

TAPPING ROUNDS

Now do 2 to 3 rounds of tapping on the 8 points:

EB	Eyebrow	This food addiction
SE	Side of Eye	This weight problem
UE	Under Eye	This addiction to food
UN	Under Nose	My obsession with food
CH	Chin	My preoccupation with food
CB	Collar Bone	This compulsion to eat
UA	Under Arm	This compulsion to binge on food
TH	Top of Head	My intense urge for food

Next we'll tap for our ability and deservingness to lose the weight. Frequently, this is a major stumbling block to our weight loss efforts.

SET UP

KC Even if I never get over this food addiction, I deeply and completely love and accept myself.

KC   Even if I never lose this weight, I choose to deeply and completely love and accept myself anyway.

KC   Even if I never stop eating compulsively for the rest of my life, I choose to love and accept myself anyway.

TAPPING ROUNDS (2-3)

EB	Eyebrow	I may never get over my compulsive eating
SE	Side of Eye	I'm afraid I may never lose this weight
UE	Under Eye	I don't feel like I can do it
UN	Under Nose	I'm ashamed that I have this food addiction
CH	Chin	I'm a food addict
CB	Collar Bone	I'm a sugar addict
UA	Under Arm	I'm a carb addict
TH	Top of Head	I'm a binge eater

SET UP

KC   Even though I don't deserve to lose the weight, I deeply and completely accept myself.

KC   Even though a part of me doesn't believe I deserve to lose this weight, I deeply and completely accept myself anyway.

KC   Even though I don't feel like I deserve to get over this food addiction, I choose to deeply and completely love, accept and honor myself anyway.

TAPPING ROUNDS (2-3)

EB	Eyebrow	I don't deserve to lose this weight
SE	Side of Eye	I'm not perfect
UE	Under Eye	I don't deserve to be happy
UN	Under Nose	I don't believe I deserve to be thin
CH	Chin	I can't get over this food addiction
CB	Collar Bone	I have to be fat
UA	Under Arm	I don't deserve to get over this addiction
TH	Top of Head	It's who I am

SET UP

KC   Even though I eat to stuff my emotions, I deeply and completely accept and forgive myself.

KC   Even though I use food to soothe my feelings, I deeply and completely accept myself anyway.

KC   Even though I use food to comfort myself, I choose to deeply and completely love, accept and forgive myself anyway.

TAPPING ROUNDS (2-3)

EB	Eyebrow	I eat to soothe my emotions
SE	Side of Eye	I eat so I don't have to feel
UE	Under Eye	I eat to calm myself
UN	Under Nose	I eat when I'm bored
CH	Chin	I eat when I'm sad
CB	Collar Bone	I eat when I'm angry
UA	Under Arm	I eat when I'm lonely
TH	Top of Head	I eat when I'm depressed

By now you should be feeling a little bit more at ease tackling your compulsive eating problem. You may be feeling a bit more confident about your ability to overcome your problem too. And that's what we want. You should also be feeling a bit calmer. You might be feeling more relaxed, and open to exploring your feelings. You might even feel hopeful about releasing your food addiction and having a better life. That's terrific! In the next section, you'll be tapping for your favorite addictive substances.

Tapping For Specific Cravings

Now that you've tapped for the problem in general terms, you've broken down some of the initial barriers you may have to ending your addiction. Now it's time to begin getting more specific. If you're anything like I was, you have some definite "go to" comfort foods. My drug of choice was anything bready or cheesy. Others may prefer sweets or chocolate for their fix. But for me, pasta, cheese and bread were favorites of mine. And I believed that macaroni and cheese was quite possibly the perfect food. The combination of warm, doughy carbs and fatty cheeses went straight to my brain's comfort center. Everything was right with the world once I sat down with my bowl of Fettuccine Alfredo. Until I went back for seconds. And thirds. Then the awful over-fullness, guilt and recriminations would begin. It was a painful cycle of bingeing, shame, anxiety - then bingeing again to control the anxiety.

As a compulsive eater, these cravings are probably all too familiar to you. There are likely definite foods that you turn to for comfort. They're the ones you want when you're feeling stressed, or sad, or even when you want to celebrate or reward yourself. Now it's time to address these specific food cravings. Take a moment to think about your favorite foods.

What foods are you most like to binge on? What foods do you have to have each day just to get by? What foods give you the most comfort when you think about eating them? What foods are you powerless to resist if you see or smell them? List them here:

_____

_____

_____

_____

_____

Ask yourself what you love most about these particular foods. How do they feel in your mouth? Do they remind you of any times from your childhood? List any thoughts or memories you may have about why you love your favorite foods here:

_____

_____

_____

_____

_____

How would you feel if you couldn't have these foods anymore?

Was that last question a little painful? It was for me. But don't worry. By the end of this program, you'll no longer look at food as your only source of comfort and reward. But right now, on a scale of 1 to 10, how anxious would you be if you couldn't have these foods? I'll bet it's pretty close to a 10!

Next we're going to tap for your specific food cravings. Insert the name of your favorite foods in the blanks provided. Feel free to add any descriptive adjectives you'd like to make the phrase more personal, or the food even more appealing. In my workshops, I ask the participants to bring their favorite junk food with them, to help facilitate the process. You can do the same if you wish. Just set your favorite food in front of you and try to build up an intense craving by thinking about how wonderful it would be to eat it. Mentally describe for yourself what you love about the food. Imagine the flavor, smell and texture of it.

When you've built up a good craving, begin tapping with the suggested set up phrases below. Remember to complete each set up phrase with "I deeply and completely love and accept myself", repeat the set up 3 times, and do at least 2 to 3 tapping rounds before moving on to the next set up phrase. Feel free to riff on the tapping rounds by using your own words, ideas or insights. Let's start with:

KC   Even though I have these cravings, and I really love the way _____ tastes, I completely love and accept myself.

KC   Even though I crave _____, I deeply and profoundly love and accept myself.

KC   Even though I have cravings to eat _____ all the time, I deeply and completely love and accept myself anyway.

EB	Eyebrow	These cravings for _____
SE	Side of Eye	My deep desire for _____
UE	Under Eye	This strong urge to have _____
UN	Under Nose	This need to eat _____
CH	Chin	I want some very badly
CB	Collar Bone	I need to have it now
UA	Under Arm	Nothing else will do
TH	Top of Head	I simply must have _____

KC   Even though I can't resist _____, I deeply and profoundly love and accept myself.

KC   Even though eating _____ is the only thing that makes me feel better, I deeply and completely love and accept myself anyway.

KC Even though I have to have _____, I choose to deeply and completely love and accept myself anyway.

EB	Eyebrow	Even though I'm powerless to resist _____
SE	Side of Eye	I have to have it
UE	Under Eye	It's the only thing that make me feel better
UN	Under Nose	_____ is my drug
CH	Chin	_____ is my tranquilizer
CB	Collar Bone	_____ is my reward
UA	Under Arm	_____ relaxes me
TH	Top of Head	_____ is the only thing that calms me down

KC Even though I eat _____ to feel better, because I love how it makes me feel, I completely accept and forgive myself anyway.

KC Even though I use _____ to self-medicate, I deeply and profoundly love and accept myself.

KC Even though I reach for _____ to calm myself, I choose to deeply and completely love and accept myself anyway.

EB	Eyebrow	_____ calms me down
SE	Side of Eye	_____ relaxes me
UE	Under Eye	_____ cheers me up
UN	Under Nose	_____ is my Prozac
CH	Chin	Food is my drug
CB	Collar Bone	Food is my only friend
UA	Under Arm	My food is always there for me
TH	Top of Head	Food is my comfort

KC   Even though I don't want to give up my favorite foods, I deeply and profoundly love and accept myself.

KC   Even though I resent having to give up my favorite foods, I deeply and profoundly love and accept myself anyway.

KC   Even though I don't want to give up _____, I choose to deeply and completely love and accept myself anyway.

EB   Eyebrow   I don't want to give up my food
SE   Side of Eye   You can't make me give it up
UE   Under Eye   I won't let you make me give it up
UN   Under Nose   I resent having to give up my food
CH   Chin   It makes me sad to think about giving it up
CB   Collar Bone   It makes me mad
UA   Under Arm   I'll be lost without my _____
TH   Top of Head   How will I make it through the day

Excellent work! Now take a deep breath and see if you can feel a greater sense of lightness surrounding your cravings. The urgent need to have your favorite food should be gone. You should have a more neutral feeling about it, like you could take it or leave it. In the next section we will focus on our out of control overeating behavior.

Compulsive Eating Behavior

As I shared with you earlier, my favorite comfort foods were starchy carbohydrates and cheese. Most days, breakfast wasn't a big problem for me, and I could usually eat a reasonable lunch.

The problem times for me were mid-afternoon after lunch and dinner time. In the middle of the afternoon around 2 p.m., while working at an administrative job I didn't particularly like, I would usually experience extreme boredom combined with a persistent subconscious anxiety. The only way I knew how to deal with that discomfort at the time was to reach for a starchy snack. Starches are a great drug for temporarily boosting our serotonin levels. For me, there was nothing better than gorging on a couple of fistfuls of salty, crunchy Cheezit crackers to take the edge off. Problem was, after the momentary oral gratification of the crackers wore off, the boredom and anxiety were still there.

It got even worse after I got home from a long day of work. For dinner, I would make a giant potful of pasta and load it up with sauce, and parmesan cheese. Then I'd plop down in front of the television to eat it. I did this to numb my feelings of anxiety, boredom and general disappointment with my life until it was bedtime. After my first, usually huge helping of pasta, I would feel totally full and bloated, but the pleasure centers in my brain were crying out for more. My taste buds still needed to feel the glorious, cheesy flavor and buttery texture of the pasta, and so I would eat until the food was all gone. That could have meant 2 or 3 helpings in all. Afterward, my feelings of disgust and guilt were overpowering.

Compulsive eating behavior is driven by intense emotions. Right now, overeating is probably your primary mechanism for stress relief in your life. Unfortunately, this same compulsive behavior creates even more stress and guilt, thereby perpetuating the cycle (We'll talk about some other ways to relax, besides eating, in Chapter 10). And there are most likely times during your day when the struggle is the hardest. In this section, you'll address your own out of control eating style and begin to explore its roots.

Ask yourself the following questions:

What types of foods are your biggest downfall? Do you normally crave sweets, chocolate or carbohydrates to get your fix? Why do you think you choose these particular foods?

_____

_____

_____

_____

_____

How many times a day do you binge? Do you binge every day? If not, why do you think that is?

_____

_____

_____

_____

_____

_____

What times of day do you normally engage in compulsive or binge eating? What are you typically doing when you feel the craving coming on? Why do you think you do it at these times especially?

_____

_____

_____

_____

Now let's begin tapping for your out of control eating behavior. Remember to tap on the set up 3 times, concluding with "I deeply and completely love and accept myself', and do a minimum of 3 rounds of tapping. Tap first for the suggested set up phrases below. As you tap on them, make any adjustments you'd like in order to make them better fit your own personal situation. You'll have an opportunity afterwards to tap for your answers to the questions above.

KC Even though my eating is out of control, I deeply and completely love and accept myself.

KC Even though I'm powerless over food, I deeply and profoundly love and accept myself.

KC Even though I'm a food addict, I choose to completely love, accept and forgive myself anyway.

EB	Eyebrow	Even though I'm obsessed with food
SE	Side of Eye	Even though I'm a carbohydrate addict because they make me feel _____
UE	Under Eye	I'm addicted to sugar because it tastes _____
UN	Under Nose	I have an enormous appetite
CH	Chin	I'm a closet eater
CB	Collar Bone	I'm embarrassed that I'm a binge eater
UA	Under arm	I have an urge to eat whenever I see food
TH	Top of Head	I have a craving whenever I smell food

EB	Eyebrow	I use food to soothe myself
SE	Side of Eye	I eat to calm down when I'm anxious
UE	Under Eye	I use food to self-medicate
UN	Under Nose	I eat whenever I'm bored
CH	Chin	I eat when I'm angry
CB	Collar Bone	I eat when I'm sad and lonely
UA	Under Arm	I eat to "stuff" my feelings
TH	Top of Head	I eat to try and avoid thinking about my life

EB	Eyebrow	Even though I stuff myself
SE	Side of Eye	And I binge to the point of discomfort
UE	Under Eye	And I never know how to stop
UN	Under Nose	I eat until I'm overfull
CH	Chin	If some is good, a lot is better
CB	Collar Bone	This overeating
UA	Under Arm	This compulsive eating
TH	Top of Head	This unhealthy addiction

KC   Even though I eat even when I'm not really hungry, I deeply and completely love and accept myself.

KC Even though my eating behavior is compulsive, I deeply and completely love and accept myself anyway.

KC Even though my overeating is unhealthy, I choose to deeply and completely love, accept, and forgive myself now.

EB	Eyebrow	Even though I crave carbs/sweets in the afternoon/at night
SE	Side of Eye	Even though I always want _____ every afternoon/at night
UE	Under Eye	Even though I binge at night
UN	Under Nose	I eat after work to unwind
CH	Chin	I sit in front of the television and stuff myself
CB	Collar Bone	Even though I overeat in front of the television
UA	Under Arm	It's the only way I can take my mind off of work
TH	Top of Head	Eating feels soothing after a long hard day at work

EB	Eyebrow	I eat when I feel overwhelmed by stress
SE	Side of Eye	I need to eat to relax and feel calm
UE	Under Eye	Stuffing myself calms me down
UN	Under Nose	I can't feel relaxed unless I'm eating
CH	Chin	I need my snacks to keep calm at work
CB	Collar Bone	I need my snacks to relieve the boredom at work
UA	Under Arm	They're my reward for the stress at work
TH	Top of Head	Eating keeps me from thinking how much I hate my job

EB	Eyebrow	Even though I want to overeat when I go out to dinner
SE	Side of Eye	I want to binge when I'm eating with friends
UE	Under Eye	And I binge whenever I socialize
UN	Under Nose	I want to taste all the wonderful food whenever I'm at a party
CH	Chin	Even though I crave _____ whenever I drink
CB	Collar Bone	Even though when I have a drink, I want to binge on _____
UA	Under Arm	When I have some carbs, I need more carbs
TH	Top of Head	I can't have "just a little"

KC Even though I have this food addiction, I still choose to accept myself with kindness and compassion.

KC Even though I have this compulsive eating problem, I can accept that this is just where I am right now.

KC Even though I'm overweight, I'm only human, and I've been doing the best I can and I choose to deeply and completely love, accept, and forgive myself now.

EB	Eyebrow	I accept myself with gentleness and compassion
SE	Side of Eye	I completely accept myself without judgment
UE	Under Eye	After all I'm only human
UN	Under Nose	I'm willing to see it differently
CH	Chin	I'm open to learning how to heal
CB	Collar Bone	I'm open to the possibility that I can lose the weight

| UA | Under Arm | I'm willing to accept the possibility that I can be thin |
| TH | Top of Head | I choose to learn how to love myself and be healed |

Now that you've completed the sample set ups, go back to the questions at the beginning of the chapter and use your answers to create personalized set up phrases. Your answers to those questions are very important, as they constitute some of your own personal compulsive eating triggers. For example, let's say you answered that popcorn reminds you of watching TV as a family growing up. Your set up might look something like this:

| KC | Even though the taste of popcorn reminds me of the good times as a kid, I deeply and completely love and accept myself. |

EB	Eyebrow	I love the taste of popcorn
SE	Side of Eye	Popcorn reminds me of the good times
UE	Under Eye	Popcorn is my comfort
UN	Under Nose	Eating popcorn makes me feel good
CH	Chin	Even though I crave popcorn
CB	Collar Bone	I just have to have popcorn
UA	Under Arm	Popcorn is my drug
TH	Top of Head	Eating popcorn is how I relax

Continue tapping on each of your personalized set up phrases. When you're finished, take a deep breath and relax. You've done a lot of work in this chapter and you should feel proud of your accomplishment. Take some time to rest and process your emotions before continuing on to the next chapter.

Here are some simple exercises designed to be done each day while going through the Thinstead program:

Daily Exercises

I recommend the following simple daily exercises to all of my clients. They're extremely helpful for focusing your mind on eliminating your compulsive eating behavior, as well as heading off your cravings before they get too intense.

🦋 Exercise: Tapping to Set the Tone for the Day

Each morning as you're standing in front of the mirror getting ready for the day, I suggest you do a couple rounds of tapping on:

Even if I never get over this weight problem, I deeply and completely love and accept myself.

Even if I never lose the weight, I choose to deeply and profoundly love and accept myself anyway.

You should also tap on these set up phrases before going to bed at night. This way you are programming yourself for success before going to sleep, as well as preparing yourself for the day ahead. By repeating these phrases, you're not agreeing to remain overweight, you're affirming your unconditional love for yourself – even with all your flaws. Self-acceptance is critical to your success in weight loss, as well as in life in general.

🦋 Exercise: Tapping Before Meals and Triggers

My clients are often anxious about not being able to stop eating when they sit down to a meal, or being able to resist a craving when it comes on. So I usually talk with them and help them identify what typically triggers their cravings during the day. Then I have them tap in advance of their meals, as well as before events or times which seem to be their triggers.

For Gloria, this meant tapping before she got out of her car after work, before going inside the house. Gloria had gotten into the habit of immediately cooking food the moment she got home after work, so extreme was her anxiety. She felt the need to eat the moment she walked through the door after a long hard day at a job with a boss she greatly disliked. I suggested Gloria tap while still sitting in her car in the garage for "Even though I need to eat the moment I walk in the door" and "Even though I have this anxiety". I also suggested she reprogram her habits by changing her clothes, going through her mail, and then taking her dog for a walk before cooking dinner, in order to break her pattern of having to eat immediately upon arriving home from work.

What are your own triggers? Some of the most common trigger situations for binges often include; break times at work, dinner time, after dinner in front of the TV, meeting friends at a restaurant, or going to a party. Take a minute to identify your own trigger moments, then develop your set-up and reminder phrases and tap on them just before they come up each day. For example, let's say you're an afternoon binger who loads up on candy or chocolate bars at 2:30 every day. So then after lunch, around 2:00, but before you feel a binge coming on, you would tap for something like:

KC   Even though I have to have a candy bar every afternoon to keep me calm, I deeply and completely love and accept myself.

OR

KC   Even though I have this anxiety, I deeply and profoundly love and accept myself anyway.

Note: If you feel uncomfortable tapping at your desk at work, take a restroom break and tap inside the stall. There's also a great short hand I like to use when I'm in public or driving in my car and something comes up. I simply tap on my collar bone point. Tapping this one point can be very effective at reducing stress and often looks to others like you're simply scratching an itch. Try it sometime in the car and see how it works for you.

❦ Exercise: Tapping to Reduce Cravings

Whenever you feel a craving for a particular food coming on, tap for it right then and there. Tap the craving away using the following phrases. As always, feel free to embellish or personalize the phrases to make them more meaningful to you.

KC   Even though I really want _____, I deeply and completely love and accept myself.

KC   Even though I must have _____, I deeply and completely love and accept myself.

Keep tapping on all the things you love about your favorite food until the craving goes away. If you find yourself struggling, and you end up eating one of your craving foods, between each bite, do a round of tapping on the 8 tapping points. You don't need to do the set-up phrases again, just tune into the feelings you have while you're eating. Eventually, the extreme craving you were having will subside, and you'll be able to throw the remaining food away without any difficulty.

🦋 Exercise: Tapping for Daily Upsets

Each one of us has incidents that happen during the day which affect our positive mood. Perhaps a disagreeable coworker does something that makes us angry, or maybe we get a traffic ticket on the way to work. These negative situations add additional stress to our lives and increase our desire to binge on our favorite foods.

I recommend tapping right after any negative incident to relieve any stress and tension before it accumulates. For example:

KC   Even though I got that speeding ticket, I deeply and completely accept myself.

KC   Even though I was so stupid, I deeply and completely accept myself anyway.

KC   Even though it's going to be expensive, and I don't have the money to pay for it right now, I choose to deeply and completely love and accept myself.

You get the idea. Remember to tap for all the negative thoughts and emotions you're feeling in response to the negative event. By committing to doing these simple exercises every day, you'll be able to remove the emotional stressors that cause your compulsive eating behavior even more quickly.

In the next chapter we're going to delve even deeper into your emotions. We're going to explore your childhood, family dynamics and relationships in order to release other issues which may be contributing to your compulsive eating behavior.

Chapter 5

※

Childhood Trauma And Our Need For Love

One major, if not the number one, emotional contributor to food addiction is the need for love and acceptance. When we didn't receive it as children, our need for love, affection and validation causes us to seek it elsewhere. This lack of nurturing in childhood leaves us with a hole in our soul that needs filling. Food, alcohol and drugs are just some of the ways we try to fill up this empty space inside us. As compulsive eaters, food is our drug of choice, and our one reliable source of comfort.

In this chapter, we'll be dealing with our need for love and affection, as well as the thornier issues of childhood trauma. Many people who suffer from food addiction have also experienced childhood abuse of some sort. Childhood abuse - whether physical, sexual, or simple emotional neglect – affects our lives deeply. It colors the way we look at the world, what kind of relationships we have, and who and what we ultimately become later in life. In the sections that follow, you'll be taking a look back into your childhood for any events, situations or memories which are contributing to your current food addiction problem.

At this point, you may be feeling a little apprehensive about delving into your past. The whole point of using EFT is not to cause additional pain, but rather to **gently** release our stored anxiety and emotional pain. And so it is a very useful tool for easing any apprehension you may be having at this time. It's completely understandable that a person who experienced a deep trauma like physical or sexual abuse would not be eager to go back and re-experience it. However, it is vital to go back and re-examine the emotions surrounding these memories if we want to release our compulsive eating and food addiction once and for all.

So if you have some memories in the past that you're fearful of dealing with, now is the time for you to tap for this fear. You can tap for any anticipatory fear by creating your own set up phrases that reflect your unique situation. They might look something like this:

KC   Even though I don't want to relive the memories of my childhood, I deeply and profoundly love and accept myself.

KC   Even though I'm afraid to feel the feelings about _____, I deeply and completely love and accept myself.

KC   Even though I'm afraid to think about (my father molesting me/Uncle Jim violating me/the rape/ being beaten), I deeply and completely accept myself anyway.

KC   Even though it's too painful to look at, I completely love and accept myself anyway.

EB   This fear of _____
SE   This fear of _____
UE   This fear
UN   This fear
CH   This anxiety
CB   This anxiety
UA   This remaining fear
TH   This remaining fear

Tap for your fear now. Keep doing rounds of tapping until your fear is reduced to near zero. If you find that you're unable to bring the intensity down for some reason, perform the collar bone breathing procedure for massive psychological reversal that you learned in the beginning of Chapter 4.

Once you've neutralized the fear of finally dealing with your childhood issues, now you can start identifying the emotional aspects from your childhood that are contributing to your current food addiction problem. This chapter will focus on physical and sexual abuse, as well as the general childhood emotional issues faced by most food addicts.

If the sections on abuse don't immediately seem like they pertain to you, just go ahead and read through the sections without tapping on anything that doesn't pertain to your situation. However, you may be surprised by the memories that come up as you read through those sections. Most people are able to remember times that they were punished or shamed in some way while growing up. These things are just part of the human experience. There is still plenty to learn about your own emotions by reading through those sections, as well as an important exercise I cover called the "Movie Technique".

Growing Up Hungry

It's been said that the ideas we have about the world and how it works are ingrained in us by the time we're 7 years old. If that's the case, then our family members, especially our parents, played a huge role in forming our psyche. And since they don't give out parenting handbooks to new moms and dads, your parents probably just raised you in the same manner they were raised.

And that way may not have always been the most loving way. Even though they were probably doing the best they knew how, they may have made some mistakes along the way which caused you to feel unloved, unsupported, or that you weren't good enough. Fortunately, you now have the tools you need to release these needful feelings once and for all.

In order to prepare for the next tapping section, take some time to think about your family life growing up. Answering the following questions will help you to develop your own personal list of memories to tap on. Be as thorough and descriptive as you can with your answers, so that you can use those details in your set up phrases later.

Growing up, what was your relationship like with each of your family members? How do you wish your relationship had been <u>different</u>?

Mother:

_____

_____

_____

_____

_____

_____

Father:

_____

_____

_____

_____

_____

Brother/Sister(s) Was the relationship with any one more difficult or problematic than another?

_____

_____

_____

_____

_____

Grandmother/Grandfather(s):

_____

_____

_____

_____

_____

_____

Are there any other family members whom you might have negative feelings associated with? Why?

_____

_____

_____

_____

_____

_____

What was it like for you growing up as a child? What did you learn about the relationship between adults and children?

_____

_____

_____

_____

_____

Did you experience any abuse, either physical or emotional, at the hands of a family member or other authority figure? If so, how did you cope with that abuse at the time?

_____

_____

_____

_____

_____

How did the abuse make you feel? What message did it send to you as a little child? What did this experience teach you about life and your place in the family and in the world?

_____

_____

_____

_____

_____

If you didn't experience any abuse per se, were both of your parents nurturing? Were any family members verbally abusive toward you?

_____

_____

_____

_____

_____

Those questions were probably somewhat painful to answer. Looking back, you may be a little sad to see how far from ideal your childhood really was. It's okay. After you tap on these hurtful feelings and memories you'll feel a wonderful sense of relief and freedom. If you'll notice, each one of the sentences in your answers above probably forms the basis for a perfect set up phrase. Simply by adding the words, "Even though" and "I deeply and completely love and accept myself" to your answers, you can create setup phrases that are highly personal and relevant to your current food addiction. Please take a moment and tap for all your answers to those questions before moving on.

Now before we continue tapping on our childhood memories, there is one more very important question to answer:

What are the 5 most traumatic, distressing or bothersome memories that you can recall growing up?

Try and recall as many as you can, because it's virtually guaranteed that these memories are the very ones contributing to your current problems with food. Give each memory a brief name like "the time I was locked in the closet" or "the time dad hit me with a belt" or "the time grandma called me a fat little piggy". If you can come up with more than 5, that's fine too. Because the more memories you tap on, the sooner the overarching aspect will be collapsed. There's a "generalization effect" that occurs in EFT, whereby if you tap on enough specific memories or events, the entire emotional issue will be released. So the more specific memories you can come up with, the better off you are.

85

List your 5 most traumatic or distressing memories here:

1._____

2._____

3._____

4._____

5._____

Do you recall any additional memories? List them here:

_____

_____

_____

_____

_____

The memories that you've just identified are literally the key to unlocking your food addiction. This will probably be the most difficult chapter in the book, since it deals with painful emotions that most people have spent their entire life trying to avoid. But if you stick with it, and diligently tap on each of the painful memories you've unearthed, you will release the pain and be well on your way to healing your food addiction once and for all!

In the following sections, we will begin tapping for any physical abuse, sexual abuse, emotional neglect or unfulfilled need for affection that we experienced growing up. Remember, if you didn't experience any physical or sexual abuse in your childhood, you may skip over the set up phrases that don't pertain to your situation. However, keep in mind that most children are at some point spanked, hit, or have something withheld in order to punish them. You may still have issues related to one of more of these instances. Also, it's important to read through the sections on physical and emotional abuse regardless, in order to learn the specific techniques I will be covering.

The section on emotional neglect is extraordinarily important for all food addicts. Because even if you didn't experience any physical or sexual abuse, chances are your emotional needs were not properly met as a child, or you wouldn't be trying to fill yourself up with food now. Our compulsive eating behavior is our way of saying to the world that we are literally "starving" for love and affection. So I invite you to pay extremely close attention to that section.

Childhood Abuse

Estimates for the percentage of children who are victims of childhood abuse are difficult to quantify. Definitions of what constitutes abuse vary, but four basic subcategories are generally recognized by experts. They are neglect, physical abuse, sexual abuse and psychological or emotional abuse. The Children's Bureau of the US Department of Health and Human Services issued their Child Maltreatment 2009 report which covered reports of abuse to Child Protective Services. These reports are estimated to encompass a population of 6 million children. This staggering number reflects only those incidents reported to CPS. It is both logical and reasonable to assume that additional numbers of children suffer from incidents of abuse that go entirely unreported.

A large percentage of victims of childhood abuse go on to become food addicts. I see many in my work. Nadia came to see me because she was very depressed and unhappy with how her life was going. During our session, I observed that she didn't exhibit much in the way of emotion, either positive or negative. We discussed her childhood, and she shared that she and her brother had been routinely beaten by their father, and explained that her mother had stood by and let the abuse continue.

When I asked her if she'd like to release the pain surrounding that experience, she said she didn't have any feelings about the abuse. She felt she had dealt with it and moved on. But judging from her overall lack of emotion and disconnectedness from her own feelings, I felt that she had just dissociated from them as her way of coping. In my experience, many victims of abuse learn to "turn off their emotions" as a way to protect themselves from the pain. In the process, they learn to turn off every emotion, including the positive ones, like happiness and joy.

So in an effort to help Nadia get in touch with her emotions again, I asked her if she felt it was fair that she had been abused. She admitted that it wasn't fair, and so I asked her if we could tap on that. She agreed and so she tapped for: "It's not fair that I was abused", "Why did it have to happen to me?", "I shouldn't have had to go through that", "Even though I don't have any real feelings about it", "Even though I can't feel anything", "I've walled myself up", "I can't feel anymore", etc. After tapping for a while, she began to realize the emotional toll the abuse had

88

actually taken on her life, and Nadia began sobbing almost uncontrollably.

Since her emotions were surfacing in such an intense way, I had her re-adjust her focus to her crying instead of the overwhelming feelings she was experiencing. She began to tap for "this crying", "these tears", "these tears of pain", "these tears of sadness", "these cleansing tears", "these healing tears", "It's safe for me to feel now", "It feels good to let go", "It's safe to feel my feelings now". After a bit, she stopped crying. We were then able to go back and tap for her disconnectedness from her feelings, and ultimately for the abuse itself. When I saw her a few weeks later, Nadia had done a complete 180. She was smiling and bubbly, and even had plans to take her first European vacation.

Like Nadia, many victims of child abuse have learned to dissociate from their emotions as a self-protective measure to help them get through life. If you find that you have a hard time mustering up any feelings surrounding your own abuse, somewhere along the way you probably felt you had to repress your feelings just to survive. It's completely understandable that you would protect yourself in that way. If you feel that your emotions may be stunted, I would suggest you tap for that before trying to access the feelings surrounding your childhood experiences. Here are some set ups and reminder phrases you might try:

KC   Even though I can't seem to feel any emotions surrounding my abuse, I deeply and completely love and accept myself.

KC   Even though I had to shut off my emotions to survive, I deeply and completely love and accept myself anyway.

KC   Even though it wasn't safe to feel my emotions, so I turned them off, I choose to completely love and accept myself anyway.

EB   I don't have any feelings
SE   I lost my feelings
UE   I can't feel anything
UN   I refuse to feel my feelings
CH   What if it was safe for me to feel
CB   What if I did feel my emotions
UA   It's safe for me to feel and express my emotions
TH   I can experience my feelings and let them go

The emotions that surface when we revisit episodes of childhood abuse can sometimes be very strong. I've found that most of the time they can be very effectively reduced and released by doing tapping rounds while they are being experienced. But if you find at any time that you are experiencing waves of emotion that you feel are too intense, you should **shift your attention to the physical sensations** occurring in your body at that moment, and tap while tuning in to them.

This could mean focusing on your tears, or even your breathing, while tapping on the 8 tapping points. Tuning in to your body will cause you to shift focus away from whatever emotion you had been experiencing and calm you down very rapidly. In the example above, Nadia shifted her focus to her tears, which helped to bring down her level of emotion quickly.

Even though memories of abuse can be some of the most difficult to face, if you are a survivor, this chapter will help you to release the trauma, sadness, and anger produced by your childhood experiences. It may seem impossible if you are new to EFT, but I assure you that you can get to a neutral place when you think back on your abuse, if you tap on enough aspects.

Now you'll begin tapping on the 5 (or more) most distressing memories you identified earlier as the doorway to your healing. You'll be using a highly effective EFT technique called the Movie Technique, which was developed to specifically address and gently dissolve particularly traumatic memories.

The Movie Technique

The Movie Technique involves taking a specific event in your life, making a brief movie out of it, and playing it back in your head. The Movie Technique helps to accomplish the goal of being specific because movies are by their very nature specific. As you run the movie in your head, you will recall many details about the event, such as sights, smells, feelings, details about the other people in the scenario and what exactly they did or said.

Here's how it's done. First select the particular traumatic memory that you wish to work on. Try and start with the most troublesome or intense one on your list. Let's say you were routinely physically abused by your father. You would select a particular time that he abused you that stands out in your memory. Preferably it should be something that lasts a few minutes, not days. The movie needs to be highly specific and short enough to easily re-run in your mind in just a few minutes.

Next give the movie a title. It should be something short, like "the time dad hit me for spilling juice on the rug" or "the basement incident". It should be something specific that describes and sums up the event briefly in your mind. If you can, run this movie in your mind, trying to feel all the feelings you experienced while living through it. Assess your current emotional intensity and assign it a number on the scale from 1 to 10. If that's too scary for you, try guessing what number you would give it IF you were to run it through your mind. Often the numbers will be the same anyway, and this may be a safer way for you to estimate its intensity. Is it a 10? An 8? A 7?

Next, do a few rounds of tapping on the 8 tapping points only, (skipping the set up) for the phrase "this _____ movie" until your emotional intensity about reliving the event has been brought down to a more comfortable level. Once you have completed that, you're going to begin narrating the movie out loud to yourself. Start by telling the story out loud, bit by bit, in as much detail as you can. But it's very important for you to STOP and do rounds of tapping on the 8 points at each segment of the story which causes you ANY emotional intensity whatsoever. Keep tapping on that particular segment of the story until you no longer have any intensity concerning it. Addressing each bit of intensity immediately, as it surfaces, allows us to get through the whole event without being totally overwhelmed by emotion.

When you're done narrating and tapping on the story segments, re-run the entire movie again and see if any further intensity pops up. Perhaps new details come to light that create more emotion, or perhaps the quality of your emotion changes to something a little different than it was before. Tap for any of the newly emerging emotion. Re-run the movie again, and continue narrating and tapping until all the emotional charge is gone from the event.

When you can run the movie through your mind's eye and get a zero level of intensity, you know you have collapsed it and you can move on to the next movie memory. Continue doing the movie technique on all the specific memories that you identified earlier, until your level of intensity drops to zero. Just tap on the 8 points without doing the set up. Go ahead and do the movie technique now for each one of the most distressing memories you identified earlier, before moving on to the next section.

How did that feel to relive each one of those experiences and be able to release the emotions tied to those events? By now, when you think back on them, you should be feeling very neutral about the incidents themselves. Even so, you may still have some feelings surrounding having had to go through them. Here are a few sample set ups and reminder phrases you can tap on relating to physical abuse. Be sure to personalize them using your own words and experiences.

KC   Even though I was terrified of _____, I deeply and completely love and accept myself.

KC   Even though I was scared of _____, I deeply and completely love and accept myself.

KC   Even though I felt _____, I deeply and completely love and accept myself.

KC   Even though _____, I deeply and completely love and accept myself anyway.

EB   Even though I wanted to run and hide
SE   Even though it was their job to protect me
UE   Even though they were supposed to love me
UN   I endured so much that I shouldn't have had to
CH   It wasn't fair that I was robbed of my childhood
CB   Even though I knew crying would only make it worse
UA   So I hid my emotions
TH   I learned I had to stuff my feelings

When I think back on those experiences of abuse, I think:

_____

_____

_____

_____

Now write out some set ups based on your thoughts and feelings listed above:

KC   Even   though   _____, I   deeply   and
      completely love and accept myself.

KC   Even   though   _____, I   deeply   and
      completely love and accept myself.

KC   Even   though   _____, I   deeply   and
      profoundly love and accept myself.

KC   Even   though   _____, I   deeply   and
       profoundly love and accept myself.

KC   Even   though   _____, I   deeply   and
       completely love and accept myself anyway.

Don't forget to use reminder phrases and tap for as many rounds as you feel you need to. The reminders can be exactly the same for each point, or you can mix them up as you prefer. There's no wrong way to do it. Make sure you tap on every thought that comes up concerning your experiences of abuse and keep tapping until you feel calm and neutral about them before moving on.

Sexual Abuse

For some food addicts, their childhood memories are even more traumatic because they involve sexual abuse. According to the Rape Victims Advocacy Program, in the United States, 1 out of every 3 females and 1 out of 5 males have been victims of sexual abuse before the age of 18 years. In fact, a National Institute of Justice study released in 1997 reported that of the 22.3 million children in the U.S. between the ages of 12 and 17 years, approximately 1.8 million were victims of sexual assault or sexual abuse. Female child sexual abuse victims are at an even greater risk for developing eating disorders and other substance addictions later on in life. They are also three times more likely to suffer from other psychiatric disorders. Those statistics are staggering. With numbers like that, it's very likely that childhood or adolescent sexual abuse has touched our lives, or the lives of those we love, in some way.

Sexual abuse carries with it profound and lasting effects that shape who we ultimately become, or don't become, in later life. The sad truth is that the effects of childhood sexual abuse don't stop when the abuse is over. Some of the more common long term effects often include depression, anxiety disorders and phobias, addiction problems (including food, alcohol and cutting behaviors), sexual dysfunction, dissociative disorders and even post traumatic stress. If you've been carrying around this heavy emotional burden, then it's very important for you to finally address these emotions and release the power they have over you.

Even if some areas of your life are currently healthy and productive, you may have a deep well of untouched emotions that can cause problems in other areas of your life, like food addiction. For example, survivors often have a hard time building healthy relationships due to a mistrust of others, and a general sense of betrayal. They also frequently experience extreme anxiety or low self-esteem which drives their urge to binge on food and/or alcohol in order to numb their feelings.

In this section we'll take a look at some of the emotions that are commonly experienced by many survivors of sexual abuse, and begin releasing them one by one. If you're feeling a little anxiety about reliving some of the experiences in your childhood, don't worry. You'll be able to tap before starting to revisit these experiences, as well as during, to bring your emotional intensity down. In fact, by the time you're done tapping, you'll begin to feel quite neutral about them. I promise.

To start with, here is a list of some of the symptoms that victims of sexual abuse typically report experiencing. Do any of them seem familiar to you?

Guilt/Shame

Do you feel like damaged goods?

Do you feel guilty or ashamed? Do you feel dirty?

Do you blame yourself in some way? Do you think you somehow brought it upon yourself?

Betrayal

Do you feel betrayed by the perpetrator, or members of the opposite sex in general?

Do you feel betrayed by your body because you felt some pleasure as a result of your own natural physiological response?

Did you try and tell your parents or another adult? Did she/he/they believe you? Was anything done to punish the perpetrator?

Do you have difficulty trusting others?

Anxiety

Do you suffer from anxiety or panic attacks?

Do you feel helpless and afraid most of the time?

Do you suffer from any phobias?

Are you afraid to sleep alone, have bad dreams or night terrors?

Do you eat, drink or cut yourself to dull the anxiety?

Depression

Are you sad and lonely?

Do you have suicidal thoughts?

Are you unable to enjoy the slightest things?

Do you feel like your wants, needs and feelings don't matter?

Anger

Do you feel angry that your human rights were violated?

Do you feel like your childhood was stolen from you?

Are you angry that nothing was done to stop the perpetrator?

Do your feelings of anger and rage impact your life and relationships?

Addictions

Do you use food, alcohol or other substances to self-medicate in order to feel better?

Do you binge in secret?

Do you cut yourself, pull your hair, or engage in other self-mutilation behaviors to quell your anxiety?

Poor Relationships

Do you have few friends?

Do you have difficulty forming close relationships?

Do you constantly seek approval? Do you seek love from inappropriate partners?

Do you have issues with trust and intimacy in your romantic relationships?

Do you have issues with poor boundaries, issues with abandonment, or are you a "control freak"?

Do you have a pattern of re-victimization?

Do you avoid sex altogether, or have you developed a "promiscuous" lifestyle as a way to exert your power over members of the opposite sex?

Do you have trouble saying "no"?

Do you find excuses not to have to go out?

Do you self-isolate so that you don't have to interact with others?

Do you feel "different" from other people? Do you feel marked or "scarred"?

Body Issues

Do you have a poor body image?

Do you wear excess, or unflattering clothing as body armor for "protection" or otherwise make yourself invisible to members of the opposite sex?

Do you have any physical symptoms left over from childhood, like gagging or difficulty swallowing?

Do you suffer from any type of chronic illnesses, such as chronic fatigue syndrome or achy joints?

As you read over the list above, how many of the symptoms are you currently experiencing? You may want to make a mental note or even write down which ones felt true for you. They will make excellent set up phrases for tapping later. Also think about what emotions came up as you read the list. Did it all seem so unfair? Did you become sadder or angrier that your life has been affected in those ways? Were you unaware that you had some of those issues until you saw it on paper? These thoughts and emotions about your childhood are the very keys that will lead you out of darkness and back into the sunlight.

Releasing The Pain Once And For All

Helen grew up in a large family of 7 children, 5 of whom were boys. She had been sexually abused by her brother Frank beginning at age 5. One day her brother and a male cousin had taken Helen into the shed in her backyard and were taking turns assaulting her. All of a sudden the children heard Helen's mother approaching the shed. When she discovered them, she dragged them all into the house and began beating the 3 of them with a belt. Helen said, "I was terrified and in pain. I was so sad and confused. I didn't even know what I had done wrong. After that, Frank would come into my room and rape me almost every night. I was terrified of the sound of footsteps in the hall. My mother was supposed to protect me, but she didn't."

Understandably, Helen felt betrayed by her brother and cousin. But she also felt betrayed by her mother - the one person she thought she could turn to for love and security. Instead, her mother completely ignored her plea for protection, and even punished Helen for what her attackers did. It's easy to see why Helen was having trouble dealing with her emotions and had problems with binge eating. She was trying to fill up the deep hole in her heart that was crying out for the love and affection she should have received from her parents, but didn't.

In working with Helen, I suggested we do the movie technique on the shed incident, as well as a few other major incidents she could recall. But she was a little afraid, so before we started the movie technique, I had her tap on her apprehension about reliving the events from her childhood. She tapped on, "Even though I'm afraid to relive the abuse", "Even though I don't want to feel those feelings again", and "Even though I'm afraid to open up and be vulnerable again". After that, she calmed down a bit, and was ready to begin honing in on the specifics of the abuse.

I had her select 3 of the most vivid and emotional incidents and do the movie technique on those, since quite often the generalization effect will then engage and the emotional release will extend out to all the other incidents. Helen also tapped for; the terror and confusion she felt during the rapes, the physical pain of the abuse, the powerlessness she felt, of being afraid to go to sleep at night, the fear of the footsteps coming down the hall, being beaten by her mother, the confusion of being punished the same as her attackers, being betrayed by her mother, and all the other specific sights, smells, sounds and sensations she felt while the abuse was going on.

While running through her movies, I had her stop whenever she felt like the emotions were too intense, and continue tapping without moving on, until she felt them ease up. After her intensity came down, she would then pick up where she left off in the movie. After she was done with the first incident, I had her run the second and third movies in the same fashion. There were definitely some cleansing tears along the way, but I made sure Helen re-ran each movie and tapped until she could no longer feel an emotional intensity regarding them. When we were finished, I asked her how she felt as she looked at those memories again. She said, "When I re-run the movie, there's no emotion there. It's like it's happening to someone else. I just don't feel those emotions anymore. I don't even feel like crying. I finally feel free of it for the first time!"

Now It's Your Turn

The fear, guilt and shame that victims of sexual abuse carry inside can be overwhelming. If you've experienced the painful emotional aftermath of sexual abuse yourself, you will be able to heal that hurt in this section. As always, if you happen to be experiencing any anticipatory anxiety about dealing with your memories of abuse, you can do a little pre-tapping for your fear:

KC   Even though I'm afraid to feel the feelings again, I deeply and completely love and accept myself.

KC   Even though I don't want to think about _____, I deeply and profoundly love and accept myself.

KC   Even though I'm afraid I'll die if I really feel those feelings, I deeply and profoundly love and accept myself anyway.

With rounds of:

this fear...
this remaining fear..

When you've brought your anxiety down, now you're ready to deal with the individual memories themselves using the movie technique you learned earlier. First select your 5 most distressing memories related to your abuse and give the movie of each of them a brief and descriptive name. List them here by their brief movie name:

1._____

2._____

3._____

4._____

5._____

If you can, run the first movie in your mind, and assess your current emotional intensity by assigning it a number on a scale from 1 to 10. If you can't do that just yet, just guess what number you would give it **IF** you were to run it through your mind. The number will still be a very accurate assessment of your emotional intensity. Next, do a few rounds of tapping on the 8 tapping points for the phrase "this _____ movie" until your emotional intensity has been brought down.

Once you have completed that, begin narrating the movie out loud to yourself, stopping to do rounds of tapping on the 8 points at each segment of the story which causes you ANY emotional intensity whatsoever. Keep tapping on each particular segment of the story until you no longer have any intensity concerning it. Do as many rounds of tapping as is required to bring your level of intensity down. Take as much time as you need. There's no need to rush.

When you're done narrating and tapping on each of the story segments, re-run the entire movie again and see if any further intensity pops up. Notice any new details that come to light, or any change in the quality of your emotions. Tap for any new information or insights. When you're done, re-run the movie again, and make sure all the emotional charge is gone from the event. If not, just start the process over and let any new memories associated with the event come forth that might also need to be tapped on.

When you can run the movie and get a zero level of intensity, you know you've released it and you can move on to the next movie. Continue doing the movie technique on all the specific memories that you identified, until your level of intensity drops to zero for each one of your movies.

When you feel you're done running your movies, take a deep breath and assess how you feel. Do you feel lighter? Clearer? Tears or yawning are always good indicators that you have had some significant release. Now when you look back on the abuse, how do you feel? Do you feel fairly neutral, or do you still have sadness or anger? Hopefully by now, the lingering trauma surrounding your abuse has been neutralized. However, you may still have feelings about the people in your life, and how they handled the situation, or how the abuse has affected your life up to this point.

Complete the following sentences with as many emotions as you can think of:

I'm angry that _____

I'm angry that _____

I'm sad that _____

I'm sad that _____

I feel betrayed by_____

I feel betrayed by_____

It's not fair that _____

It's not fair that _____

I needed _____

I needed _____

I wanted _____

I wanted _____

I feel guilty that _____

I'm ashamed that _____

I wish _____

I should have _____

Now take each one of these phrases and turn it into set up phrase, and tap on each one doing at least 2 to 3 rounds of tapping like so:

KC   Even though I'm angry that my innocence was taken away from me, I deeply and completely love and accept myself.

KC   Even though I needed to be loved and protected, but
_____ ignored my abuse, I deeply and completely
love and accept myself.

Remember to do 2, 3 or more tapping rounds, until your intensity
has been brought down to zero. Continue tapping on all the
emotions you can think of surrounding your abuse. Here are some
common emotions expressed by abuse survivors you may find
helpful to tap on:

Even though _____ was supposed to love and protect me

Even though I'm angry that my innocence was stolen

Even though I'm sad that my childhood was destroyed

Even though _____ betrayed me

Even though my mother/father/parents didn't protect me

Even though _____ didn't believe me

Even though my parents should have loved and protected me

Even though I'm angry that nothing was done to _____

Even though I needed to be loved, and I didn't get it

Even though I was punished even though I was the victim

Even though I told _____ and they didn't help me

Even though I've suffered so much pain

Even though the abuse ruined my life

Even though my life would have been much different if the abuse hadn't happened

Even though it wasn't fair what happened to me

Even though I feel dirty

Even though I feel like damaged goods

Even though I feel ashamed and scarred

Even though I can't have normal relationships

Even though I can't open up and trust people

Even though I can't trust men/women

Even though the memories of the abuse hold me back

Even though I'm afraid all the time

Even though I'm so sad and lonely

Even though I hate my body because of it

Even though I can't stand sex because of my abuse

Even though I feel betrayed by my body, because I felt some pleasure while it was happening

Even though I stuff my feelings with food because of the abuse

Even though I have this food addiction because of the abuse

Even though I'm overweight because of the abuse

These are just some examples. It's really important for you to put your feelings into your own words when tapping. Continue tapping until you can't think of any more negative emotions to tap on.

Weight As Protection

Victims of rape, molestation and incest frequently use their excess weight as a protective barrier to keep them safe from potential predators. The extra pounds they carry on their body can often be a sort of shield or armor used for protection. If you've been the victim of physical abuse, you may subconsciously think that keeping a layer of padding will protect you from further assault. Or in the case of sexual abuse, your excess weight can be a way of protecting yourself from unwanted advances and even more violation. For some of us, it may not feel safe to lose weight. Losing the weight would leave us without our protection.

If losing your excess weight feels a little scary, you may have some internal resistance to losing weight. That subconscious resistance can impede your weight loss efforts. So to break down that barrier, we need to tap for the fear of losing weight. Here are some set up and reminder phrases you can use. Feel free to personalize them, or even add some of your own.

KC   Even though it feels scary to lose weight and be without my padding, I deeply and completely love and accept myself.

KC   Even though I'm afraid to be without my armor, I deeply and completely love and accept myself anyway.

KC   Even though I don't want to lose my protection, I choose to deeply and completely love and accept myself anyway.

EB   I'm afraid to be thin
SE   My weight protects me
UE   It keeps me from being hurt
UN   My weight keeps me from being harassed
CH   It keeps me from being violated
CB   My weight keeps men away from me
UA   My extra padding is my armor
TH   It's my protection, and I don't want to lose it

EB   What if I let it go
SE   What if I allowed myself to lose weight
UE   I think I could let it go
UN   I choose to let the weight go
CH   I choose to feel safe about losing weight
CB   I choose to feel safe and confident without the weight
UA   I can allow myself to feel safe now
TH   I choose to feel safe while losing weight

Congratulations for sticking with it and tackling the most difficult emotions you will ever have to face. You deserve to be proud of all your hard work and what you've achieved so far. Hopefully by now, you should be getting some distance from the emotions that surround your abuse and you're ready to move forward. Next we're going to examine our need for love that wasn't completely fulfilled while growing up.

Emotional Neglect: Starving for Affection

Even if you didn't experience of any type of physical abuse while growing up, chances are that your parents were not fully spiritually enlightened beings who raised you in an atmosphere of unconditional love. There may have been times in your childhood when you felt less than loved and supported. As a result, today as an adult you could still be "starving for affection". Most food addicts have deep issues relating to one or both parents. They often feel like they weren't loved in the way they needed, or were constantly criticized, or were told that they were stupid or "not good enough". Everything a food addict does is a reflection of this insatiable need for parental love and affection. And while our parents probably loved us in the way they best knew how, chances are it was not in the way we needed to receive it, or we wouldn't be trying to fill ourselves up with food.

Ariel grew up without a father, and her mother was controlling and emotionally cold. In our sessions together, it occurred to Ariel that she was using food as more than just a way to soothe the emotional emptiness from her childhood. She was also using it as a way to punish her mother, as a kind of giant "Screw you! I'm in control now." It became clear that she was very angry with her mother and was using food not only to ease years of emotional

111

pain, rejection and abandonment, but also as a way to assert some kind of control over her own life and wrest it away from her domineering mother. Ariel's story underscores just how complex and nuanced our feelings toward our parents can be. Often, there can be a mixture of sadness, anger and loneliness underlying our need for the love and affection we never got. This section will help you focus in on the unfulfilled need for love, attention and acceptance which is driving your food addiction.

As you think back on your childhood, how was your relationship with your parents? Did you feel valued, loved and supported at all times? Or did you feel invisible? Did you have to "perform" in order to be loved? Did your parents punish you by not speaking to you, or did they withdraw their love when you did something they didn't like? Was there any sibling rivalry in your family? Was anyone in your family an alcoholic or into drugs? If so, it's very probable that somewhere along the way, you learned that you weren't good enough just the way you are.

And when that happens to us in childhood, we try to make up for it as adults by attempting to fill our hearts up using food. It's not our parents' fault. They were just doing the best they knew how. They more than likely raised you the same way they were raised. It's a rare and lucky child that grows up with an unconditionally loving set of parents. Nevertheless, lack of love and affection has a tremendous effect on our emotional development.

Janie was the eldest of two daughters. Her mother was emotionally distant with her, while her sister Jennifer was the favorite of the two. Her sister was considered the pretty one and received the most attention from her mother. But Janie could never do anything without being criticized. Janie came to see me for her food addiction and depression. During our session she

112

realized she was trying to make up for the lack of love and affection she received in childhood by turning to food for comfort. During our talks, she also came to realize that she was a "people pleaser" and had a tendency to acquiesce to everyone else's wants and desires. She had a pattern of putting other people's needs before her own. As a result, she put the fulfillment of her own dreams on permanent hold. She felt like she wasn't really living. You may recognize a little of yourself in Janie's story. That's not unusual, since many food addicts grow up trying to perform up to others' expectations in order to be loved.

Ever since Emma could remember, food was an important part of her family life. As a child, every time they got a good report card at school, she and her brother were given candy. And although she couldn't remember many instances in her childhood when her parents encouraged her or listened to her, she knew she could count on a captive audience around the dinner table. So for Emma, food represented both reward and nurturing. When she realized this, she said, "You know, I can't really recall the last time my mother initiated kissing or hugging me, or told me I was good. I realize that she let the food do the talking. Food was my reward, my comfort, my way of receiving the nurturing I really needed from her growing up. No wonder I love food so much!" For most food addicts, food has come to take the place of the love and parental affection they didn't get while growing up. And until we heal this deep void within us, we are destined to remain addicted to food.

Sometimes the lack of love we feel comes from a neglectful or completely absent parent. Tricia's father left her family when she was just 8 years old, never to return. Even before he left Tricia's mother, he had been an emotionally absent, self-centered kind of man. He was only concerned with his own life and never considered other family members' wants or needs as being important. The abandonment that Tricia felt at her father's leaving was almost overwhelming. So Tricia tapped on "Even though my father never paid attention to me", "Even though he never noticed me", "I just wanted his love and attention", "But he just LEFT", "He just abandoned me", "He abandoned us", "He just threw me away like garbage", "Like I was nothing", "My heart was broken", "I'm still trying to win his love", "But I'm never going to get it" and "So I'm trying to fill myself up with love by overeating".

When she was done tapping, I could see her visible relief. When I spoke to her a week or so later, she said she was no longer bingeing, and had even broken it off with a man she had been seeing because he was too "emotionally unavailable". She said that she realized that she deserved more from a relationship and wanted to stop trying to "win" a man's love.

Here are some questions designed to get you thinking about your childhood, your family life, and the role food plays in your life today. Take as much time as you need to fully explore your feelings.

Thinking back on your childhood, would you say your parents were very demonstrative with their love and affection? Or were you more likely to get some kind of treat like candy or cookies, if you did something right?

_____

_____

_____

_____

_____

Can you easily remember moments of being hugged, kissed or told you were smart, or is it hard to recall the good times?

_____

_____

_____

_____

_____

Did either of your parents take pride in your accomplishments? Did they foster your talents and abilities? Or did they always seem to put you down? Are you in touch with your own dreams and desires today?

_____

_____

_____

_____

_____

What are some of the meanest things you can remember anyone saying to you growing up? Try and list as many things as you can.

_____

_____

_____

_____

_____

If your parents weren't very nurturing, how did you go about trying to win their love and affection?

_____

_____

_____

_____

Growing up, did you feel like you had to perform in order to be accepted? How were you punished when you fell short of perfection? Were you ignored or frozen out? Were you shamed? What did that tell you about love and how to get it?

_____

_____

_____

_____

_____

What meaning did food have in your house growing up? Nurturing? Security? Celebration? Reward? Did any of your other family members exhibit unhealthy behaviors regarding food, like bingeing or hoarding, or trying to get to desserts first?

_____

_____

_____

_____

_____

How do you think having the family you had has affected you now as an adult? What attitudes and beliefs about life did you learn from your family? Think about the beliefs you currently hold about love, relationships, trust, success, money, your body, your skills and abilities, etc. Use an additional pad of paper if you need to.

_____

_____

_____

_____

_____

_____

Using all the insights you gained from answering the questions above, create some set up phrases for yourself below (use additional sheets of paper if you need to) and tap on them.

Even though _____,
I deeply and completely love and accept myself.

Even though _____,
I deeply and completely love and accept myself.

Even though _____,
I deeply and completely love and accept myself.

Even though _____,
I deeply and completely love and accept myself.

Even though _____,
I deeply and completely love and accept myself.

Even though _____,
I deeply and completely love and accept myself.

Here are some sample set ups which are representative of typical underlying issues experienced by most food addicts. I recommend that you tap on them, using your own preferred wording, while adding in other thoughts and emotions as they come up.

KC   Even though I'm still "hungry" for love and affection, I deeply and completely love and accept myself.

KC   Even though I'm "starving" for love and attention, I deeply and profoundly love and accept myself.

KC   Even though I'm sad that didn't receive the love I wanted from you in the way I wanted, and I probably never will, I choose to love and honor myself anyway.

EB   I didn't feel loved by you
SE   You didn't know how to show me you loved me
UE   I needed to be told that I mattered, and that I was precious
UN   I just wanted to be loved for who I am
CH   You didn't love me the way I needed to be loved
CB   I'm still trying to get that love today, but I can't
UA   To this day, you still don't know how to show your love
TH   I'll probably never get the love I need from you

EB	I didn't get what I needed
SE	I probably won't ever get the love I needed
UE	What if I loved myself instead
UN	What if I gave myself the compassion I needed
CH	I deserve to be loved and understood
CB	I choose to feel loved and nurtured
UA	I choose to feel loved and accepted
TH	I choose to be whole and happy

KC   Even though I'm sad that I never felt heard or understood by you, I deeply and completely love and accept myself.

KC   Even though whatever I did as a child wasn't good enough for you, I deeply and profoundly love and accept myself anyway.

KC   Even though I'm angry that I never got any recognition or praise when I did something right, I choose to deeply and completely love and accept myself anyway.

EB	I never felt good enough
SE	Everything I did got criticized
UE	You never approved of me or what I did
UN	I felt like I was "bad"
CH	I felt unworthy
CB	I just wanted to be loved for who I am
UA	I was a child and I deserved to be loved
TH	I deserve to be loved now

EB	I was just a child and I deserved love
SE	You were my parent and you should have loved me
UE	It was your job to love me
UN	I deserve to be loved
CH	I deserve to feel loved and accepted
CB	I choose to feel loved and supported now
UA	I choose to feel loved and accepted for who I am
TH	I choose to experience love and happiness

KC   Even though I'm sad that I never got the attention I deserved, I deeply and completely love and accept myself.

KC   Even though you didn't pay attention to me, I deeply and profoundly love and accept myself anyway.

KC   Even though I felt like I didn't matter, I choose to deeply and completely love and accept myself anyway.

EB	No one paid attention to me
SE	No one cared about what I wanted
UE	I never felt like I mattered
UN	Nobody cared how I felt
CH	I felt invisible
CB	My wants and needs were ignored
UA	So I learned to put everyone else first
TH	My needs are always pushed aside

EB	Even though I can't accept that I'm not ever going to get the attention I want from her/him/them
SE	Even though my weight gives me negative attention, otherwise they ignore me
UE	I need to hang onto this weight to get attention, otherwise I'm invisible
UN	I've spent my whole life trying to win their approval
CH	I'm still trying to please them, but it never works
CB	I'm still trying to prove myself every day
UA	I shouldn't have to be perfect to deserve love
TH	I choose to see that I don't have to please them

EB	I now choose to please myself
SE	I choose to honor my own wants and desires
UE	I choose to know that I deserve love
UN	I choose to completely accept myself
CH	I deserve to feel loved and accepted
CB	I choose to love and approve of myself
UA	I choose to freely express my desires
TH	I choose to honor myself and my feelings

Siblings

Parents are not the only family members that food addicts can have issues with. Siblings can also be a source of subconscious emotional turmoil. It's inevitable in every family with multiple children that the tenor of the relationship a parent has with each child will be different. Sometimes it's painfully clear who the "favorite child" is of the bunch. This can leave the non-favorite children with some emotional baggage, as well as cause tension and sibling rivalries within the family dynamic.

Lauren had memories of her older sister Beth pinching her, pulling her hair, and even trying to scald her in the bath tub with hot water as a child. The rivalry and resentment on the part of Beth started when Lauren was born and continued on into adulthood. Beth had been an only child up until Lauren was born, and she harbored massive resentment toward Lauren for taking her parents' attention away. Lauren was deeply hurt by Beth's attitude and behavior, so I had her tap on "Even though Beth hates me", "Even though I remember Beth pinching me and pulling my hair", "Even though I remember Beth trying to scald me in the bathtub", "Beth hates me and tried to hurt me", "I have to be less than, to try and make Beth love me", "It hurts my feelings that Beth doesn't love me" and "But there's nothing I can do to make Beth love me". After a while, Lauren yawned, and I could tell she was feeling more relaxed and had released some emotion. I asked her how she felt, and she said, "That icky feeling in the pit of my stomach is gone. I feel like I can breathe deeper now too!"

Are there any tensions among the siblings in your own family? If so, where does that come from? Does one of you resent the other for something that was done or said? Do you have difficulty communicating with each other now?

List your feelings about your siblings here and then tap for any hurts, resentments or regrets that you can think of:

_____

_____

_____

_____

_____

Even though _____,
I deeply and completely love and accept myself.

Even though _____,
I deeply and completely love and accept myself.

Even though _____,
I deeply and completely love and accept myself.

Even though _____,
I deeply and completely love and accept myself.

Even though _____,
I deeply and completely love and accept myself.

Spouses

It's very common for us to become involved with, or marry someone with a personality type that is similar to one of our parents. This re-creates the experience of trying to win the approval of our parent all over again. We do this because it feels familiar and comfortable somehow. Unfortunately, it can also lead to a repetitive cycle of needing to win love, affection and approval from our mate. And because our love relationships are so intimate, our partners have the ability to wound us emotionally in deeply hurtful ways.

Lucy came to see me for her food addiction, but it soon became apparent that she was having problems in her marriage as well. She and her husband had not had sex for over a year, and they seemed to have great difficulty communicating. The two of them had clearly grown apart. Lucy felt unloved and unimportant in her marriage. To release her hurt at the loss of her husband's love and affection, she tapped on "I feel so lonely", "I miss my husband's affection", "I miss us being close", "We don't communicate anymore", "We're like strangers", "I feel rejected", "I feel like I'm unimportant", "I feel angry when he doesn't listen to me", "I feel like I don't matter", and 'Even though I'm starving for affection, I choose to love and comfort and nurture myself".

After about 20 minutes of tapping for the sadness, anger and frustration she felt in her marriage, Lucy was starting to feel better. She also understood why she had been eating so much "comfort food". She had been trying to fill herself up with the love she was missing from her husband. After our session, I told Lucy that she should keep tapping whenever she felt a craving coming on, whenever a bad memory popped up, or whenever she felt any anxiety, anger or sadness.

At her next appointment, Lucy said she was feeling much better about her life and had been able to keep her bingeing under control. She said she even felt more hopeful about making progress in her marriage. Apparently, the improvements Lucy was making in her own life, and the shift in her energy, were having an effect on her husband. He was becoming curious about what she was doing and began asking her questions. The two of them were now communicating a bit more, and Lucy was optimistic that things would get better between them.

Have you noticed any changes in your own eating behavior during your marriage/relationship? Did something happen to cause that? How do you feel about your spouse? How does he/she feel about you? Do you feel loved, supported and understood? What do you wish were different about your relationship?

_____

_____

_____

_____

_____

Now tap for each feeling and insight that came up.

Even though _____,
I deeply and completely love and accept myself.

Even though _____,
I deeply and completely love and accept myself.

Even though _____,
I deeply and completely love and accept myself.

Even though _____,
I deeply and completely love and accept myself.

Even though _____,
I deeply and completely love and accept myself.

Even though _____,
I deeply and completely love and accept myself.

Congratulations! You've just completed what is undoubtedly the most difficult chapter in the entire book. Issues surrounding childhood trauma, love and affection, family and relationships are the most foundational to food addiction, as well as some of the hardest for us to deal with. You deserve a tremendous amount of credit for loving yourself enough to improve your life. Certainly by now you should be feeling relief from the sadness and pain left over from your childhood. To further increase the emotional gains you've made, here are two extraordinarily helpful exercises I believe everyone should try.

🦋 Exercise: Write A Healing Letter

One exercise that I've found to be extremely healing is writing a letter to someone from our childhood that we still have issues with today. This could be one or both parents, a perpetrator of abuse, or even God. First write a letter to this individual explaining your feelings, and how deeply their actions affected you. Write everything you can possibly think of. The object is to have your complete say. You should write it exactly how you feel, and not candy coat it, because this person will never read your letter. It is only for you.

When you're done, re-read through your letter and tap for each sentence, or point you made, that brings up emotion for you. Tap until you feel calm and peaceful. When you're done, you will write a second letter. This letter will be **from** this individual to you. You will be writing from the viewpoint of this other person, explaining why they behaved as they did. It is my experience that this letter is an extremely powerful one. One of my clients wrote a letter to God, and through writing a response letter back, she was able to overcome her panic attacks almost immediately.

The response letter should prove to be very healing for you, but if you experience any additional negative emotion, of course you should tap for it. I recommend doing this exercise for everyone in your life that you have issues with or find challenging!

🦋 Exercise: Peeling The Onion

Next is what I consider to be the most powerful exercise in the entire book. In fact, it's so valuable that I've done it multiple times myself. Each time I run through it, I find that more and more information comes up which I missed the previous time. In EFT it's called the Personal Peace Process. But I like to call it "Peeling the Onion", because it's tremendously effective at peeling away the layers of emotional hurt that we carry resulting from the negative events and situations that have occurred in our lives.

In the Personal Peace Process, we try and identify every experience, situation or event in our life that if we had to do it all over again, we would choose to **skip**. These can be experiences where something happened or someone did something you did not like, or something that you did that maybe you wish you hadn't. Anything that made you feel sad, angry, scared, guilty or ashamed is fair game.

For the purposes of this exercise, no event is too small to be tapped on. So if someone took your lunch at school in the third grade, or hit you over the head with a book on the school bus, it qualifies! We are in the business here of scooping out every bad feeling we've ever had. Often it helps to call more incidents to mind when we visualize our lives chronologically. This exercise is so powerful that sometimes my clients make astounding progress from this one exercise alone!

Start by getting comfortable, close your eyes and take a few deep breaths. Now begin by running a movie (if you're more visual) or taking an inventory of your life beginning at birth. Can you remember your birth? Was it a difficult delivery? Was the umbilical cord wrapped around your neck or was it a breach birth? If so tap for that. Can you remember anything from your infancy? Tap for anything that may come up.

Next visualize your childhood. Is there anything you remember from being a toddler? Did someone smack your hand for taking a cookie? Were you spanked for doing something "bad"? Was there abuse? Or neglect? How were you treated at school? Were you bullied or teased? Did your teacher embarrass you in front of the class because you got a math problem wrong? Did you steal some candy from the dime store, or anything else which you now regret? Remember every detail and tap for those experiences and tap for how they made you feel.

Next visualize your adolescence. How did you get along with your parents? How were you treated by your friends and classmates? How did your teachers treat you? Were you popular or not? Were there any especially embarrassing or terrifying events at school? Did you do anything of which you are now ashamed, or that you feel bad about? How do you wish your teenage years had been different? Tap on every negative situation that comes up and how it made you feel.

Now examine your adult life. Are there any experiences or relationships that you'd just as soon have skipped over? Were there any illnesses (yours or others') that touched your life? How about any financial problems? Has your life turned out the way you wanted? Do you have any regrets? Tap on each situation, event or emotion, until you feel a profound sense of relaxation and relief.

This is one exercise that really has no end. You may be going about your daily life, perhaps standing at the sink doing dishes, and some old forgotten memory will pop up. Take the opportunity to stop and tap on it right then. I find that each time I review my life chronologically in this way, new memories pop up that I hadn't thought of before. As you continue to tap on negative memories that surface, you'll be peeling still more layers of the emotional onion that keeps you from living your best, most fulfilling life!

Chapter 6

The Other Emotions Behind Food Addiction

In the realm of food addiction and compulsive eating we tend to encounter the same emotional themes over and over. The most common aspects to the problem of food addiction (or addiction to any other substance for that matter) besides the issues of abuse and lack of parental affection, are deprivation, loss, anxiety, anger, resentment, guilt, and low self-esteem. In this chapter we will begin addressing some of these other major emotional components driving our out of control eating behavior.

Deprivation

In my work with clients, I've found that the theme of deprivation is a huge one for compulsive overeaters. We eat because we are trying to make up for what we missed out on in our childhood. We eat to prove that we are in control, and that no one can push us around. The idea of not being able to have our favorite food brings on a cascade of deprivation thoughts. How will we live without our favorite foods? How will we deal with the stress of everyday life without them? We resist the idea of giving them up to our very core. However, in order to effectively release ourselves from the bondage of food addiction and compulsive eating, this feeling of deprivation must be addressed.

Renee came to see me for her food addiction and we began to talk about her childhood. I could see that she had a highly restrictive childhood growing up and a very controlling mother. Though admittedly their family didn't have a lot of money, whenever she wanted something, be it a toy or afternoon treat, her mother always told her no. Renee grew up very frustrated, and found no joy in her life. As a child, Renee was rarely allowed to have anything she desired, so as an adult she had stopped trying to excel at anything, or have any dreams for her future. She had learned that it was no use; she couldn't have what she wanted anyway, so why bother. The one area in which she could exercise her power though, was over food. When it came to food, she was in control. She could eat whatever she wanted, whenever she wanted - even to the detriment of her health. Sometimes, like Renee, we eat to exercise control over our own lives because we weren't able to as children.

In preparation for this next round of tapping, I want you to imagine that you can no longer have your favorite foods. Say out loud to yourself, "I have to give up my favorite candy/cookies/chips." How does that make you feel? Do you feel panicky and anxious? Imagine being at lunch with your friends and not being able to have your favorite dish? Do you feel angry? Do you feel sad? Do you feel resentful? Do you feel deprived? In my experience it's pretty likely that you do. In the spaces below, create your own set up phrases by filling in the blanks:

Even though I can't stand the idea of giving up _____, I deeply and completely love and accept myself.

Even though I will feel _____ if I can't have my _____, I deeply and completely accept myself.

Even though I don't want to give up my _____, I deeply and completely accept myself.

EB   Even though I'll lose the one thing I can rebel with

SE   I don't really want to stop eating my favorite foods

UE   I'm afraid I'll have to give up my main form of comfort

UN   Even though I'll feel deprived if I can't have my_____

CH   I'm angry that I am being forced to give up _____

CB   Even though I'm afraid of being deprived

UA   Even though I feel grief when I think of giving up _____

TH   Even though I'll feel deeply deprived if I have to give it up

KC   Even though I'm feeling a lot of lack in my life, I deeply and completely love and accept myself.

KC   Even though I feel deeply deprived, I deeply and completely love and accept myself and my feelings.

KC   Even though I'm afraid I'll feel even more deprived if I give up my favorite food, I choose to completely love and accept myself anyway.

EB   Even though I never get what I really want

SE   I could never have what I wanted as a child

UE   Mom/dad never let me have what I wanted

UN   I don't want to give up the one enjoyable thing in my life

CH   Even though I refuse to go without my favorite food

CB   I deserve to have my treats and don't want to give them up

UA   But I'm afraid of having to give up my favorite food

TH   I refuse to give up my favorite food

EB   Even though I hate being told what to do

SE   I hate being told what I can and can't have

UE   I couldn't wait to grow up so I could have and do whatever I wanted

UN   Eating sweets feels like a reward

CH   My snacks are my way of rewarding myself

CB   Eating is my way of being in control

UA   I don't want to give up my control

TH   Even though I don't want to feel deprived

EB   I'll feel resentful and totally deprived if I can't have my snacks

SE   Even though I'm afraid there will never be enough

UE   There's never enough for me

UN   Even though I'll never be enough for my mother

CH   Even though there was never enough love growing up

CB   But I can choose to feel there is enough for me

UA   I choose to feel I am enough

TH   I choose to feel whole and complete

Feel free to write out any other set ups you'd like, that express your feelings about giving up your favorite foods and tap on them.

Overeating as a Form of Control

Many of my clients use overeating as their way of asserting the control they didn't have as a child. Often times, one or more of their parents were highly controlling, restrictive or domineering, and seldom let them have what they wanted. Other times, they had an extremely chaotic childhood, where nothing could be counted on to remain stable. This is especially true of households with an addict or an abuser in the parental role. Could you be using your eating as a giant "screw you" directed at someone? Are you using food as a way to finally have what YOU want for a change? Is eating the one form of control you have over your life? Does your desire for control extend to other areas of your life, turning you into a control freak?

Explore your thoughts on the subject of control and write them down here:

_____

_____

_____

_____

Using your thoughts above, create your own set up phrases and tap on them now. Here are some others you might find helpful to tap on.

Even though eating what I want is my only form of control in life

Even though people have tried to control me my entire life

Even though they're still trying to control me now

Even though I overeat as a way to take control back in my life

Even though I feel resentful over not having control

Even though my overeating is a giant screw you to _____ and everyone who tried to control me

Even though I am afraid of being deprived again if I can't have my favorite foods anymore

Even though I had no control as a child

Even though as a child my needs didn't count

Even though I was supposed to be seen and not heard

Even though my home life was chaotic

Even though my home life and my parents were unstable

Even though my father/mother could go off at any minute

Even though I was afraid most of the time because I never knew what was going to happen next

Even though I never had control as a child, I choose to be in control now.

Even though I never had control as a child, I choose to realize I'm in control of how much I eat now. I can choose to have whatever I want, and as much or as little as I want. I now choose to take charge and exercise control over my life.

Fear and Anxiety

Another common underlying emotional cause of food addiction is fear or anxiety. This can be a fear of losing control, fear of not being good enough, fear of rejection, fear of the unknown, fear of losing someone or something – these are all real fears that many of us experience every day. But sometimes, fear can emerge from even more unusual corners of our psyche.

Kate was having trouble with her compulsive eating when she would get home from work in the evenings. As soon as she hit the door, she would take off her work clothes, put on her stretch pants and t-shirt and immediately begin eating. While she was cooking her dinner, she wouldn't even stop to put items back in the refrigerator or mixing utensils in the sink, so urgent was her need to begin eating. Although we had tapped on all the usual suspects, like lack of love and self-esteem, she still had this urgent need to eat.

When she came back for the next session, I asked her what she was feeling when she had the urgent need to eat. She was able to identify it as an anxiety. We had already tapped on her fear of her life ever getting any better, and fear of being alone, and it wasn't until we started talking about her late 20's when she told me she had suffered from panic attacks. What was unusual was that her panic attacks only occurred at night and woke her out of a dead sleep. They were also often accompanied by horrible, apocalyptic nightmares. We talked some more and she revealed that she had grown up as a Catholic, during the 1970's when they would frequently do air raid drills at her elementary school and the children would get under their desks for protection against bombs.

As we talked it became clear that subconsciously, Kate still held distinct fears of both God and nuclear war. (It's not uncommon for us to view God like a parent. It's also interesting to note that we tend to ascribe the same qualities our parents had to the Creator.) So I had her tap on the aspects of "I'm afraid that God will send me to hell", "I'm afraid of total nuclear annihilation", "I'm afraid of being destroyed" and a few others. As she was tapping, I could see Kate visibly relax. We were successful in bringing her fear down to zero, and she was excited to see what would happen when she returned home from work the next day.

She called me late that next evening to tell me how happy she was that she came home from work and did not experience the overwhelming anxiety and compulsion to immediately eat. In fact, she was able to do a few chores around the house before preparing her dinner. And when she did eat, she only had one helping. She didn't feel the need to go back and make more food. She was ecstatic. I kept in contact with Kate over the next few weeks, and she had already lost a few pounds, began walking in the evenings with her neighbor and even joined a tennis class two nights a week. She said she felt as if she had entered a new chapter of her life.

Kate's story underscores the importance of digging until we find "what's really eating us". Sometimes it can be something even more exotic or unusual than we first imagine. In order to find out what fears you may have lurking beneath your food addiction, ask yourself the following questions.

What are you thinking about when you feel an intense craving come on? Are you thinking about work, and how much you hate your job? Are you thinking about your bills and debts? Worrying about your children or other family members? What is it you think you might be trying to avoid feeling by eating?

_____

_____

_____

_____

_____

_____

Turn your answers above into set ups and tap on them. Do several rounds on each until you feel calm and peaceful. Here are some other possible set up phrases for you to work with. See if any of them resonate with you:

Even though I eat when I'm bored

Even though I eat when I'm angry

Even though I eat when I'm lonely

Even though I hate my job/boss

Even though I wish my life was different

Even though I feel pressure to be responsible

Even though I'm carrying the weight of the world

Even though I worry about my children

Even though I worry about my finances and how I'm going to pay the bills

Even though I worry about my health

Even though I worry about dying

Even though I worry about _____

Even though I'm afraid _____

Even though I am convinced that _____

Even though I feel desperate about _____

Even though I'm nervous about everything

Even though I eat because I'm overwhelmed by stress

Even though I can't seem to relax unless I eat

Even though I need to eat to feel calm and relaxed

Even though stuffing myself feels soothing after a long day

As always, don't forget to tap on any other thoughts that occurred to you while tapping on the above set ups.

Panic Attacks

It's not uncommon for the same fear and anxiety which drives our eating behavior to also cause panic attacks. Fortunately, EFT works very quickly and powerfully to eliminate anxiety. Because tapping on our anxiety enables us to communicate directly with our amygdala, it can rapidly short circuit the brain's fear response. Tapping on our underlying fears, like we did in the exercise above, will help remove the triggers of our panic attacks. If we find the proper combination of aspects, panic attacks can be eliminated completely.

But even if we haven't yet gotten to the root cause of our panic attacks, EFT can be used in the moment while we are having an attack to help calm us down. If you happen to feel one coming on, take a moment to stop and tune into the bodily sensations you are experiencing. Notice your breath, heartbeat, any pain or other troubling sensations you're having. Here are some set ups you can use when you feel the onset of an attack:

Even though I have this extreme fear and anxiety

Even though my heart is racing and I feel like I'll die of a heart attack

Even though I have this chest pain

Even though I have this squeezing chest pain

Even though I'm afraid my heart will stop

Even though I feel like I am going to die

141

Even though I feel dizzy

Even though I feel like I'll pass out

Even though I feel like I am going to lose my bowels

Even though I feel like I have to escape

Even though I feel so much stress inside of me

Even though I feel overwhelmed

Even though I feel really scared

Even though I am afraid I'm dying every time I _____

Even though I'm afraid I am going to die early of _____

Even though I'm afraid I might have _____

Even though I worry about _____

Even though I worry about how I will _____

Even though I don't ever feel safe and healthy

Even though my mind is working overtime to keep me safe, I can choose to allow it to relax now.

Even though my mind is overreacting trying to protect me, I now choose to allow it to be calm and peaceful.

Panic Pre-Tapping

You can also tap in advance of any potentially anxiety provoking situation to prevent an attack from coming on like so:

Even though I'm afraid of having a panic attack whenever I _____

Even though I'm so afraid I'll have a panic attack when I _____

Even though I'm afraid to _____ because I might have an attack

Even though I'm afraid of this fear

Even though I'm afraid I'll pass out

Even though I'm afraid I'll make a spectacle of myself

Even though I'm afraid people will stare

Even though I'm afraid people will judge me

Tap for any other insights you had, or other fears you may have about having a panic attack in public. In my work with panic attack sufferers, I've found that tapping on the "fear of the fear" can be very effective.

Guilt and Shame

When we struggle with compulsive overeating, there is often a significant undercurrent of guilt and shame. These two emotions are especially destructive because the stress of suppressing them just causes more bingeing. We feel ashamed because we feel out of control of our own actions. We feel weak and worthless. We may even have done something in our past which causes us great shame. If we hope to release ourselves forever from the grip of these limiting emotions, we must learn to forgive ourselves for our failings. After all, we're only human and all people make mistakes sometimes in their lives. Ask yourself:

As you look at your life at this moment, how do you feel about your eating behavior? How do you feel about your weight?

_____

_____

_____

_____

_____

Do you have any guilt or shame left over from childhood? If so, what specifically? (Note: Shame is often a factor where there are sexual abuse issues.)

_____

_____

_____

_____

_____

_____

If you could live your life over again, is there something you did that you wish you could undo? What is your biggest regret?

_____

_____

_____

_____

_____

Do you think of yourself as a good person? Do you think you'll be going to heaven when you die? If not, why not?

_____

_____

_____

_____

_____

That last question very important. Many of us harbor tremendous guilt over our actions, and so we feel we aren't deserving. Imagining our own death, and what will happen to us when we cross over, brings these feelings of guilt and shame sharply into focus. But these feelings of guilt and shame are deeply destructive to our happiness and also contribute to our compulsive eating. It's time now to finally unburden ourselves and start tapping on the issues of guilt and shame.

Take all the thoughts and feelings that you uncovered from answering the questions above and turn them into set up and reminder phrases. Tap on them all until you're feeling calm and peaceful, then continue with the set ups and reminders below.

KC   Even though I hate myself for overeating

KC   Even though I feel guilty when I overeat

KC   Even though I feel guilty about being overweight

EB   Even though I overeat because I don't love myself
SE   Even though I hate myself for overeating
UE   I feel guilty when I overeat
UN   I feel guilty about being overweight
CH   I want to be able to forgive myself for eating when I'm sad, bored, or lonely
CB   I want to forgive myself for eating when I'm not really hungry
UA   I choose to forgive myself for overeating
TH   I choose to forgive myself now

KC   Even though I'm ashamed that I can't control my eating

KC   Even though I'm disgusted with myself

KC   Even though I can't believe I let myself get this fat

EB   Even though I'm embarrassed to admit I'm obese
SE   I'm ashamed that I let myself get this fat
UE   I'm ashamed of my body
UN   Even though I eat to avoid my feelings
CH   I use food to soothe myself
CB   I overeat to hurt myself
UA   I overeat to hide myself
TH   I binge because I think I'm worthless

KC   Even though I was shamed for eating too much as a child

KC   Even though I was criticized for being fat

KC   Even though I judge and criticize myself for being fat

EB   Even though I was shamed for eating too much
SE   Even though _____ criticized me for how and what I ate
UE   Even though _____ criticized me for being overweight
UN   I wasn't accepted for who I was
CH   Even though I felt ashamed of my body and how fat I was
CB   I forgive myself for overeating
UA   I forgive myself for being overweight
TH   I can choose to let it all go now

147

KC   Even though I still feel guilty about _____ (what I did), I deeply and completely accept and forgive myself.

KC   Even though I'm afraid to forgive myself for _____ (what I did), I was just doing the best I knew how at the time and I choose to love and forgive myself.

KC   Even though a part of me feels like I need to punish myself for what I did, I choose to forgive, love and nurture myself from now on.

EB   I feel so guilty about _____
SE   I should have _____
UE   It was so bad
UN   I don't deserve to be forgiven
CH   I feel like I need to be punished
CB   That's why I keep hurting and sabotaging myself
UA   It's because I won't let myself be happy
TH   I feel like I need to keep punishing myself

EB   But I was just doing the best that I could then
SE   If I could I would do it differently now
UE   I can stop punishing myself now
UN   I choose to forgive myself
CH   I choose to let go of the guilt
CB   I can learn to forgive myself once and for all
UA   I can love and support myself now
TH   I choose to nurture myself and allow myself to be happy and peaceful

KC   Even though I feel guilt about _____

KC   Even though I feel ashamed about _____

KC   Even though I feel all this guilt and shame, I choose to deeply and profoundly love, and accept and forgive myself.

EB   Even though I feel guilty about _____
SE   Even though I punish myself by staying overweight
UE   I can stop punishing myself now
UN   I choose to forgive myself
CH   I can let go of the guilt
CB   I choose to learn to forgive myself finally
UA   I choose to learn how to love and forgive myself
TH   I choose to allow myself to be happy, healthy and peaceful

Another type of guilt that we can experience is the guilt we feel when we attempt to lose weight and other people in our lives remain heavy. This is especially true of our female loved ones, like our mothers, sisters or best friends. How do you think your mother would feel if you lost all the weight? Or your sister? Other family members and friends? How would your relationships change? Read through the set ups below, personalizing them to fit your own situation, and tap on them.

Even though I know I'll feel guilty if I lose weight and my mother/sister/friend stays overweight

Even though I feel guilty because I'll leave her behind and I might lose her love/friendship

149

Even though I'll feel guilty about being thinner than my mother/sister/friend

Even though she'll stop being my friend

Even though we might lose our bond, and no longer have anything in common

Children of Addicts

There is a particular type of guilt that is unique to the children of alcoholics and drug addicts. Anyone who grew up in a family of addiction knows what I'm talking about. Adult children of alcoholics or addicts often suffer from feelings of not being "good enough". They feel this way because they internalized the idea that they weren't "good enough" to be able to keep their parent(s) from drinking or using, as if somehow it was their fault.

Sometimes children of alcoholics reject alcohol so as not to be like their parents, but turn to food as a socially acceptable form of addiction. The deep guilt they harbor inside needs to be addressed so that their addiction can be healed once and for all. If alcohol or drug addiction was part of your family life, the following questions are meant to help you get in touch with how growing up with an addict affected your life.

If you had to deal with a family member who was a drinker/user, how did that make you feel?

_____

_____

_____

_____

_____

How did having an addict in the family affect your life? Do you feel angry that your childhood was stolen from you? Did you have too much responsibility for a child? Were you in a constant state of fear or readiness?

_____

_____

_____

_____

_____

What behaviors were required of you just to get by, in that type of environment?

_____

_____

Many adult children of alcoholics and addicts feel the need to control their own environment at all costs because of the chaos they experienced as children growing up. What was your childhood environment like, and how do you think that has affected your adult life? Do people call you a control freak?

After answering the questions above, you may feel emotions like guilt, anger at your parents, sadness for what you lost, disappointment for how your life turned out, and many others. Make sure you fully tap on all the emotions that came up.

Here are some blank phrases to help you formulate your set ups surrounding any guilt, shame or other emotions you might still be harboring. In your set up phrase, be sure to completely love, accept and FORGIVE yourself.

Even though I couldn't _____ I deeply and completely love, accept and forgive myself.

Even though I had to _____

Even though I lost _____

Even though I'm sad that _____

Even though I feel guilty because _____

Even though I'm angry at _____

Even though they made me feel_____

Even though I'm disappointed that _____, I deeply and profoundly love, accept and forgive myself.

EB Even though I felt scared
SE I couldn't take care of myself
UE I was just a child
UN I was always lonely
CH I felt so overwhelmed
CB Even though I had too much responsibility for being a kid
UA I was never good enough to help _____ stop drinking
TH If only I had been good enough or smart enough, _____ would have stopped drinking/using for me

Before moving on to the next section, make sure you've released any lingering guilt you may have for any of your regrets, failings, past actions or deeds. Releasing guilt and shame is essential for eliminating any eating disorder.

Sadness, Grief and Loss

Some of us have suffered great losses in our lives that cause us deep sadness and grief. Whether it's a parent, grandparent, lover, best friend or a beloved pet, the loss of these wonderful beings can have a major impact on our lives. Also, there are many different types of grief. Sometimes when we endure years of health issues, that loss of joy can also create a sense of grief in our lives. Grief for what we've lost and for what might have been. No matter what caused it, grief is a powerful emotion that can lead directly to compulsive eating in order to soothe the anguish and hurt we feel inside.

Death of a Love One

Donna was struggling with compulsive eating behavior when she came to my office. She could finish off an entire bag of Oreo Doublestuffs in one evening. She felt she needed sweets to get through the day. She ate mini-donuts at her morning break, and cookies and candy bars after lunch. Then she would binge again at night when she got home from work. In our sessions, she recounted how her mother had died a long, painful death from pancreatic cancer. She had to watch her mother suffer for months until she finally died in hospice care. Donna was devastated.

She had felt powerless to help her mother during her illness, and was grieving deeply for her loss. It was clear to us both that Donna was eating to keep from feeling the painful grief of missing her mother. She tapped on "Even though I ache for the loss of my mother", "Even though I couldn't save my mother", "Even though I'll never see her again", and "Even though I'm all alone now". After we finished tapping on the loss of her mother, and her tears subsided, Donna let out a big yawn. This is usually a good sign that the issue has been resolved and that deep relaxation has set in.

I asked her how she felt about the loss of her mom, and she took a moment to go inside and check her feelings. She told me, "Of course I love my mom, but that aching feeling deep inside is gone. I don't feel like I'm going to die from the sadness and loneliness any more. The constriction around my heart and the lump in my throat are gone!" I followed up with Donna a few weeks later, and she said she felt more relaxed and hopeful. She felt like she would be okay, and that she could feel her mother's spirit around her comforting her. She no longer had the compulsion to eat to stuff down the sadness and thanked me for helping her to release her deep-seated grief.

Ask yourself the following questions to see if grief has touched your life in some way:

Have you lost a loved one in your life? Do you feel like you are "over it"?

_____

_____

_____

_____

How has it affected you in your daily life? Do you think about them a lot? Are there certain things you can't look at, or songs you can't listen to, without crying?

_____

_____

_____

_____

What do you miss most about your loved one?

_____

_____

_____

_____

What else has been lost as a result of their death? An opportunity to make amends? A weekly phone call? A shoulder to cry on? Happy holidays? Is there anything you wish you would have done or said to them before they passed?

_____

_____

_____

_____

If you haven't lost a loved one who died, is there a significant relationship that you've lost in your life? How did that affect you? What role did that relationship fill that you are missing today?

_____

_____

_____

_____

Do you maintain your relationships with other family members and friends, or have you become something of a hermit?

_____

_____

_____

_____

Tap on all your emotions surrounding the loss of your loved one, and for all the things you'll miss. Here are some other set ups you may wish to tap on:

Even though I miss _____

Even though I miss our relationship and all the things we used to do together

Even though I think I might die of loneliness

Even though I'll never see him/her again

Even though I'll never be able to touch/hug/kiss him/her again

Even though I'm afraid that holidays and birthdays will be too sad

Even though I can't watch _____ without crying

Even though I can't listen to _____ without feeling sad

Even though I feel guilty about _____

Even though I wish I could have said or done _____ before he/she died, I choose to deeply and completely love and accept myself.

Now tap on any other times that you feel are difficult, or other things you will miss without having your loved one in your life.

Death of a Dream

Another type of grief we can suffer from is the loss of a dream. Sometimes a health problem or an accident can steal the promise of our cherished desires. Whether it's a hysterectomy that crushes

158

our dream of having children, or an accident that leaves us paralyzed, or even a chronic illness like fibromyalgia that limits our ability to participate fully in our life, health problems can cause us to experience grief on a soul level. If you've been affected by a serious health issue, it's important that you tap on your feelings surrounding it to release that sadness. Think back and see what may have happened in your life to crush your hopes and dreams for the future.

When did something first die inside of you? Did some trauma or accident occur? How did your life change after that?

_____

_____

_____

_____

What else did you lose when this happened? Did you lose your sense of hope? Did you lose your sense of belonging? Your feeling of safety? Did your joy and excitement get taken from you?

_____

_____

_____

_____

When is the last time you cried? Why? What's the one thing that makes you sad?

_____

_____

_____

_____

What's your biggest regret in your life thus far?

_____

_____

_____

_____

_____

Have you suffered from any major or chronic health problems in your life? If so, how did that affect your life? Did it change your plans for the future?

_____

_____

_____

_____

_____

Tap on all of your feelings of sadness, loss and regret surrounding the loss of your cherished dreams. When you've tapped on your own set up phrases, here are some others you might want to try:

Even though I feel deep grief, and I overeat eat to stuff it down

Even though my dreams are over

Even though I'll never _____

Even though I am deeply sad about _____

Even though I'm sad that I missed out on so much

Even though I'm in pain all the time

Even though I can't take it any more

Even though I've suffered so much, and I don't want to suffer anymore

Even though my life is so hard

Even though I just want to be acknowledged for how hard it has been for me

Even though my heart aches for _____

Even though I'm so sad and I feel like God has abandoned me, I choose to deeply and profoundly love and accept myself.

Now that you've tapped for all your sadness and grief, you should feel a little expansion in your body. You may feel like your heart has opened up, or perhaps the fog in your head has cleared. That's good. You deserve to be proud of yourself for working through your grief and taking the necessary steps toward improving your life.

Boredom

These days in our society, it's all too common for people to feel depressed, sad, lonely and bored. I believe this is what is underlying the near epidemic levels of alcohol, drug, food and sex addiction being reported today. Some people are even addicted to television, video games, computers, or their smart phones. There's a pervasive sense of frustration and a lack of passion for life that seems to have invaded our culture. All of the ways we try and fill our time are just an attempt to ignore the banality of our daily life and experience a little bit of happiness.

The overwhelming majority of us profess to hating our jobs and admit to coming home, plopping down in front of the TV to switch off our brains for 4 to 5 hours every night. We are so dead inside and disconnected from what gives us joy that we often turn to having a "virtual life". Whether you're addicted to television, video games, or Ben & Jerry's, one thing's for sure – you're not really living. Henry David Thoreau is famous for saying "Most men lead lives of quiet desperation and go to the grave with their song still in them." And sadly, he's right.

Some people blame the proliferation of electronic technology for cutting us off from interacting in any meaningful way with each other. Others say it's the fault of the stifling culture of mediocrity that is the hallmark of our current K-12 educational system, where conformity is encouraged and creativity, diversity and innovation are undervalued. Whether those things are the cause, or simply that we had our dreams extinguished somewhere along the way to growing up, it's clear that we've lost our mojo.

As children we had an insatiable curiosity, and we could find hours of fascination in the smallest of things, like ladybugs, building blocks or simply banging noisily on a pot with a hefty spoon. However, now as adults, we seem to have lost our imagination, curiosity and sense of wonder. Play has taken a back seat to work. But in order to live a life of fulfillment, it's very important that we find healthy ways to stimulate our sense of creativity and exploration every day.

Nature, travel and creative hobbies are some of the best ways to satisfy our innate desire for novelty and discovery. I personally love to go hiking in the mountains. I get a deep sense of peace and connectedness from the natural beauty of the trees, sky and animal life, as well as the excitement of discovering what lies beyond that next tree or boulder. Drawing, painting, music, handicrafts and gardening are also passions for many people, giving them a feeling of purpose and anticipation when they wake up in the morning. I recommend that every person try and find a way of expressing their creativity or learning something new each day.

Depression

Depression is a pervasive feeling of hopelessness that anything will ever get better. It's as if we've been defeated by life. It is our anger turned inward on ourselves. It comes from suppressing our true selves and not living our truth. Depression also comes from not believing we can have what we want in life. And since we don't believe we can have it, we don't even bother trying. In order to free ourselves from depression, we need to release the underlying beliefs and feelings of desperation that are causing it.

Here are some useful set ups you may want to try:

KC   Even though I'm so depressed, I deeply and completely love and accept myself.

KC   Even though I feel this hopelessness, I deeply and profoundly love and accept myself.

KC   Even though I feel this deep despair, I choose to deeply and completely love and accept myself.

EB   I'm tired of feeling so sad
SE   My life sucks
UE   Even though I don't think it will ever get any better
UN   Even though I don't think it can get better
CH   Even though I'm afraid that it won't ever get any better
CB   My life hasn't turned out like I planned
UA   What's the use of trying anyway
TH   I never seem to get what I want

EB	Even though I can't remember the last time I was truly happy
SE	Even though I've lost my sense of childhood wonder
UE	And I never take the time to do anything fun
UN	And even though I've lost the ability to feel pleasure
CH	I can forgive myself for eating because I hate the way my life turned out
CB	I choose to forgive myself for eating because I don't think my life will get any better
UA	I choose to be open to being happy
TH	I choose to start feeling, hope, wonder and joy again

EB	Even though I'm so bored with my life
SE	I choose to find meaning and try new things
UE	Even though I feel stuck
UN	I choose to believe that happiness is possible for me
CH	And even though I feel like it's hopeless
CB	I choose to find a way to live my dreams
UA	I choose to nurture my talents and gifts
TH	I choose to pay attention to my wants and desires

EB	I choose to feel more optimistic about my life
SE	I choose to feel that anything is possible
UE	I'm willing to embrace the new in my life
UN	I choose to see things with new eyes
CH	I'm open to exploring my talents and abilities
CB	I choose to find a way to express myself daily
UA	I choose to find a way to use my talents to help the world
TH	I choose to live a life where I connect with and help others each day

Make sure you also tap for any insights you had while tapping on the above set up phrases.

Anger

Some people say that anger is a cancer. That may not be so far off the mark. The emotion of anger has actually been linked to many diseases. In acupuncture literature, anger is often associated with liver problems. It has also been linked to a whole host of other inflammatory diseases that include arthritis and heart disease. In fact, Dr. Judith Carroll of the University of Pittsburgh performed a study which showed that people who routinely react to challenging situations with anger instead of calm may have a much higher risk of heart disease.

As you can see, it's in our own best interest to dissolve our anger and find better ways of coping with the stressful events in our lives. EFT to the rescue! We can use EFT to dissolve our long standing angers, as well as tapping in the moment when some new situation stirs us to anger.

Even though we may realize it's in our own best interest to release our anger against someone, sometimes it isn't that easy. But forgiving someone for an offense is not about approving of their actions. It's about releasing the negative emotions you're holding inside that are harming your health. You don't have to approve of what they did, you can simply let go of carrying the anger over it around with you. Releasing anger really gives you more power because you aren't allowing another to dictate **your** mood. So for the sake of your body and peace of mind, try and forgive everyone in your life, including yourself. Begin now by asking yourself these questions:

166

Who am I unwilling to forgive? Why? Would it make a difference if you knew it was harming your health and causing possible disease?

_____

_____

_____

_____

What kinds of things, people, or behaviors really make me angry? Who really knows how to push my buttons? Why?

_____

_____

_____

_____

_____

_____

Who really has the upper hand if you're feeling angry and it's eating away at you inside? Are you really doing anything effective when you try punishing another by being angry? Could you let the anger go? Would you rather be angry, or be at peace?

_____

_____

_____

_____

_____

_____

Two of the most life limiting types of anger are anger aimed at ourselves and anger against God. They have the effect of limiting our ability to achieve our goals and sustain personal peace. Is there anything you are angry at yourself for? What do you wish you could forgive yourself for?

_____

_____

_____

_____

Are you angry at God for any reason? Do you feel as if God has let you down somehow?

_____

_____

_____

_____

Tap for all the feelings of anger you identified, until you feel no more intensity. Here are some sample set ups that you can use. Feel free to insert your answers to the above questions. Tap on every hurt and anger you can think of.

KC   Even though I'm unwilling to forgive _____ for _____, I deeply and completely love, accept and forgive myself.

KC   Even though I don't want to forgive _____ because _____, I choose to deeply and completely, love, accept and forgive myself.

KC   Even though I can never forgive _____ for what I/he/she/they did, I choose to try to forgive myself/him/her/them now.

KC   Even though I won't forgive _____ for what I/he/she/they did, I choose to try to release my anger now and find inner peace and calm.

KC   Even though I feel angry and resentful that _____, I choose to try and completely love, accept and forgive myself now.

KC   Even though I'm angry that I never seem to get what I want, I choose to listen to and honor my feelings and desires now.

KC   Even though I'm angry that my life didn't turn out the way I wanted, I choose to live differently from now on and love, accept and forgive myself.

🦋 Exercise - Making Peace with Your Enemies

Remember the Seinfeld show, and the holiday that George Costanza's dad celebrated, called Festivus? On Festivus, it was a tradition to perform what he called the "The Airing of the Grievances". As it turned out, Mr. Costanza had the right idea. The following exercise is designed to do just that – air your grievances. Here's how it works:

First, take out two sheets of paper and a pencil. On the first sheet, take your pencil and divide it into 3 columns vertically. In the first column, make a list of all the people who have ever offended you. That includes family members, significant others, friends, teachers, bosses, that surly cashier in the checkout line – whoever.

In the second column, list what it was that each of them did to offend you. Write down exactly why their actions were offensive to you. Were they being mean spirited, unkind, or two-faced? Did they lie to or about you? What kind of qualities and traits did their words or actions exemplify? For example, imagine you have a coworker in your department at your job who is constantly negative, talks about how stupid people are behind their backs, and generally bad mouths everyone. What qualities do you perceive they are exhibiting? Are they being negative, judgmental, gossipy, or two-faced? In the third column, write down some advice you might give this person.

The next step is where the exercise gains its real transformative power. Each person we meet is a mirror of ourselves in some way. The way we react to people tells us a great deal about our own patterns, perceptions, and emotional filters. In fact, it says more about us than it says about the actual behavior of the other person. And since no one can force us to feel any particular way, the negative reactions we have toward another person are really just a reflection of our own subconscious emotions and unresolved issues. We can use these same grievances we harbor against others to heal our own underlying issues and patterns. These situations are highly specific, and as we know, the more specific we are in our tapping, the more successful we will be at unraveling the underlying issue.

Next, take the second sheet of paper and divide it into 2 columns. List your own name in the left hand column. In the right hand column, you are going to list specific examples of situations or times in your life when YOU exhibited the same negative qualities or traits that you listed for each person on the first piece of paper. Doing this will put you into contact with the exact issue, feeling or memory that you most need to resolve. After completing your list of examples, you are now going to tap for each one.

So for our negative coworker in the example above, it might go something like this:

Even though I'm judgmental of other people's clothing and appearance when I am out shopping, I deeply and completely love and accept and forgive myself.

Even though I'm acting two-faced when I'm nice to Ellen and then talk about her behind her back to Megan, I now choose to deeply and completely forgive myself.

Even though I always have to be right when I argue with Don, I now choose to deeply and completely forgive myself.

Do a couple rounds of tapping for each example of you personally exhibiting that same negative quality. After you're done, go back and look at your list of people and evaluate how you feel about each one now. Your negative emotions toward each person should have subsided. If you feel a little residual emotion left for anyone, re-examine what other possible quality or trait might be causing that and repeat the exercise. By the end, you should find that you no longer harbor ill will toward the people on your list. The issues you were reacting to should be released. Now doesn't that feel freeing? Happy Festivus!

Chapter 7

Self-Esteem and Body Issues

Growing up, if we were told repeatedly that we were bad, or not good enough, it may have damaged our self-esteem. Or if our parents stopped talking to us until we apologized every time we did something wrong, we may have felt like we had to "perform" in order to be loved. As children we may have received the message that we weren't worthy somehow, or that we didn't matter.

Perhaps in our adolescence we were teased or made fun of at school. One of our classmates might have embarrassed us in front of the whole class. Even in our adult lives, we're not immune from shame and embarrassment. Our romantic relationships can also be a source of esteem-shattering, soul crushing moments. Lack of self-esteem can manifest in our lives in a number of ways such as; poor body image, perfectionism, being a people pleaser and self-sabotaging behavior, just to name a few. In this section, we tackle some of these issues and finally put them to rest. Begin by answering these questions:

Thinking back, did you feel unconditionally loved and supported as a child? If not, why not? Did you feel like you had to perform in order to be loved? Write down some concrete examples:

_____

_____

_____

_____

_____

Can you name three to five of the worst incidents or situations in your life that may possibly have injured your self-esteem?

_____

_____

_____

_____

_____

Make sure you tap for each the thoughts and feelings you just uncovered above before moving on. Here are some other sample set ups relating to the topic of self-esteem for you to tap on:

KC   Even though I feel like I'm not good enough, I deeply and completely love and accept myself.

KC   Even though I didn't feel loved enough growing up, I deeply and profoundly love and accept myself now.

KC   Even though I'm not lovable, I choose to love and accept myself and all my failings anyway.

EB   Even though I'm not good enough
SE   Even though I didn't feel loved enough
UE   Even though I'm not lovable now
UN   Even though I feel completely unlovable
CH   I'm not as good as everyone else
CB   I'm never good enough
UA   I feel like I don't fit in
TH   I feel like I don't belong

EB   Even though I wasn't enough
SE   Even though I'll never be enough
UE   Even though I feel inadequate
UN   I don't feel worthy
CH   I'm not worthy of reaching my goals
CB   Even though I see myself as fat and ugly
UA   Even though I hate my body
TH   Even though I'm full of self-loathing

KC   Even though my mother/father/_____ never really saw me for who I am, I deeply and completely love and accept myself.

KC   Even though she/he didn't really SEE me, I deeply and profoundly love and accept myself anyway.

KC   Even though she/he sometimes just saw me as a nuisance, as a child to be seen and not heard, I choose to love and accept and cherish myself anyway.

EB   Even though she/he just saw me as a nuisance and a bother

SE   Like I didn't matter

UE   Like I don't count

UN   Even though he/she/they ignored my feelings

CH   I choose to understand that she was just doing the best she knew how

CB   I choose to feel closer to her/him because we were raised the same way

UA   I choose to accept that they loved me even though they didn't know how to show it

TH   I choose to understand that they loved me even though they couldn't show me in the way I needed it

KC   Even though I feel like I can't increase my self-esteem, I now choose to accept responsibility for my feelings and actions.

KC   Even though a part of me thinks I can't do anything right, another part knows I do some things very well, and I choose to love and accept myself anyway.

KC   Even though a part of me thinks I'm stupid and I can't do anything right, the other part knows that I'm intelligent, competent and capable, and I choose to love and accept myself exactly the way that I am.

EB   Even though my childhood experiences may have contributed to the problems I have today

SE   Even though I let my self-esteem be determined by what others think

UE   Even though I've avoided being responsible for my own self-esteem

UN   I choose to see and acknowledge my own achievements

CH   I choose to feel I deserve to reach my goals

CB   I choose to believe I deserve to be thin

UA   I choose to believe I deserve to finally lose the weight

TH   I now choose to see myself as worthy of success

Perfectionism

Not feeling worthy or good enough can often lead to perfectionism. Perfectionism is about trying to make ourselves worthy and loveable through our efforts. We may even feel guilty for enjoying ourselves instead of working. We think we will be loveable if we can just be thin enough, attractive enough, smart enough, successful enough or work hard enough. But these efforts are doomed to failure from the start, because self-love and acceptance are an inside job. The pressure to be perfect brings with it an enormous amount of anxiety which acts as a powerful driver to compulsively eat.

Can you identify any areas in your life where you feel the need to be perfect? Here are some questions to think about:

If you normally wear makeup, are you comfortable with letting people see the real you without it? How about your family? Friends? Strangers? Are you able to leave the house to do errands without wearing makeup? Why?

_____

_____

_____

_____

How do you feel when you make a mistake at work? Why? What's the worst that can happen?

_____

_____

_____

_____

When you're in a group of people and you don't agree with what someone is saying, do you speak your mind? Or do you clam up, for fear they won't like you? Why do you think that is?

_____

_____

_____

_____

_____

When someone asks you for a favor and you don't want to do it, what do you tell them? Do you lie to make it easier? Why? What are you afraid of?

_____

_____

_____

_____

_____

_____

If these questions make you a little sad, it's probably because you very much want to be liked by others. You need their approval because you're still trying to win the approval you didn't receive growing up. You probably also feel like you need to look, act or be perfect to win their affection. You can begin to heal your self–

esteem now by tapping on your answers to the questions above. Tap until you feel calm and peaceful.

When you're finished, here are some more set ups you can try:

Even though everything I did was criticized as a child

Even though I feel the pressure to be perfect

Even though I have to be perfect

Even though I'm not perfect but I feel like I have to be

Even though I feel like I'm a failure

Even though I wish I could accept myself as not perfect

Even though I very much need to be liked by others

Even though I'm fat, so I'm not perfect

EB	I need to do it all perfectly
SE	I have to appear perfect
UE	I'm not okay as I am
UN	If I'm myself I won't be accepted
CH	If they really knew me they wouldn't like me
CB	I do what everyone else wants so they will love me
UA	I suppress myself to makes others like me
TH	I need other people to validate me

EB   Even though I had to perform in order to be loved
SE   Even though I never received any acknowledgement or approval when I did something good
UE   Even though I feel like a loser
UN   I feel so ordinary
CH   I feel like I haven't achieved very much in my life
CB   I'm such a failure
UA   I'll always be a failure
TH   I'll never achieve anything

EB   I'm starting to see that I don't have to be perfect to deserve love
SE   I want to believe I deserve to be happy
UE   I deserve to be heard, and to ask for what I want
UN   I choose to stand up for myself
CH   I choose to take care of my own needs
CB   I choose to believe I am worthy of happiness
UA   I choose to believe I am capable
TH   I choose to nurture my soul and honor my spirit from now on

EB   I'm okay exactly as I am
SE   I choose to validate myself
UE   I choose to learn to express my truth at all times
UN   I choose to be myself with others
CH   I choose to be true to myself
CB   I choose to allow others to see the real me
UA   I know I'm worthy of love
TH   Even though I'm not perfect, and I'm never going to be perfect, I choose to love, accept and forgive myself anyway

Remember to always treat yourself with gentleness and compassion. Because no matter where you are in your life, you are always doing the very best you know how. Try and extend to yourself the same love, compassion and understanding that you would give a small child. Your soul is made up of the same beautiful spiritual essence, and you are no less deserving of love and understanding - no matter your age, or where your life has taken you.

🦋 Exercise: A Million Thanks

When our self-esteem suffers, we tend to think and say mean things about ourselves, our bodies and our abilities. This exercise is designed to break that cycle, and give us a little vacation from self-criticism for a while. In this exercise, we're going to set some time aside to appreciate ourselves for all the hard work we do for ourselves and our family each day. It's probably best to do this exercise on a weekend since your schedule will be freer and you won't have to rush to get ready for work.

Beginning from when you arise in the morning, you're going to silently thank yourself for every tiny task you do. I mean **every** task. Even the most minute task, like washing a coffee cup. So it would sound like this in your head; "Thank you Tina for washing your face. Thank you Tina for putting on your slippers and robe. Thank you Tina for measuring the coffee. Thank you Tina for putting the coffee pot on..." You get the idea.

It may seem silly to you at first, because most of us aren't used to feeling appreciated. Especially for the small things. This exercise allows us to appreciate ourselves for all the things we do for ourselves and others every day. Try and keep this exercise going for as long as you can. It feels really good to be appreciated. In fact it may feel so good, you may want to do it more than once. Go ahead! It's a great way to train yourself to feel good about yourself just the way you are.

Body Image

Most people with weight problems have body issues of some kind. Whether it was someone who made fun of you in school, or a family member that criticized you and judged you, somehow you got the message that your body was less than adequate. And if you are anything like I was, looking in the mirror can be genuinely painful. I'd step out of the shower and quickly put on my pajamas and robe so that I didn't have to look at my naked body in the mirror. If I did catch a glimpse of myself in the mirror, all I could see was my fat stomach and cottage cheese thighs. This body image problem prevented me from having a romantic relationship for nearly ten years. I didn't feel that any man could love me, or even want to have sex with me with my body as it was. I was in my own private little hell of body shame.

If you're a female who grew up in the United States, you've literally been bombarded all your life with images from television, movies and magazines telling you that you MUST be thin to be beautiful. The media tells you that if you're not thin, you're not worthy. Just look at the models in our fashion magazines and our celebrities. They all seem to be under nourished, stick-thin waifs that could blow over in a stiff breeze. Sadly, our thin-obsessed culture has given birth to whole generations of women with eating disorders and an unhealthy relationship with food.

This media message of "thin is beautiful" not only affects women's body self image, but it also tends to shape what men in

183

this culture define as attractive. Caroline was in a relationship with a man for about 8 months, and was very much in love. She had also gained a few pounds from eating whenever and whatever her naturally slim beau ate. She was seriously considering marrying this man, when over Valentine's Day dinner he said to her: "Do you ever think a person could gain so much weight that they would no longer be attractive to their mate?" Caroline's heart was crushed by her lover's words. He had just rejected her for how her body looked. Caroline ultimately broke it off with this man, but from that moment on, she continued to gain even more weight as a mechanism to keep men away - men whom she feared would ultimately reject her if she let them get close to her. Men that she felt she could not trust with her heart.

Can you think of a time in your own life when you received the message, either implicitly or explicitly that your body was unattractive? Can you remember a time when someone rejected or shamed you about your body? Did someone send you the message that you were too fat to be beautiful? If so, you've probably internalized this harsh judgment about yourself, and continue to perpetuate it by being your own worst critic. We think all sorts of unkind things about our bodies every day. So to help release our body shame, and tap in self-acceptance, we are first going to do some mirror work.

🦋 Exercise: Mirror Work

Stand in front of your mirror either naked or in your underwear (a full length mirror is best, so you can see all of you). This part may be a little uncomfortable at first, but it's very important. If you wish, you can do a few rounds of tapping for "Even though I'm scared to look at myself in the mirror" or "Even though I'm terrified to look at my body naked", to bring your intensity down.

184

If there are tears along the way, don't worry. They are part of the healing process, and you can tap silently while you're crying to bring your intensity down some more, until you feel like you can continue.

In this exercise you will examine every inch of your body beginning with the top of your head down to your feet. Look at every part of your body and say exactly what you feel about it. Don't hold back. It may feel a little foreign at first, because most of us haven't given ourselves permission to talk about our bodies this way out loud. You're going to tap on every critical thought you have ever had about your body. As you're taking inventory of your body, think about the words you use to describe your body part, and frame your set up phrase using those same exact words. Each time you encounter a body part you don't like, do your set up phrases and tap a minimum of 2 to 3 rounds on that body part – more if you feel like you need it.

It will go something like this:

Even though my hair is so frizzy and ugly, I deeply and profoundly love and accept all of myself.

Even though my eyes are too close together

Even though I have a turkey neck

Even though my breasts look like two deflated balloons

Even though my stomach is so fat and bulgy

Even though my butt is so dimply and gross

185

Even though I have all this cellulite

Even though I have these ugly stretch marks

Keep tapping for all your perceived bodily flaws. Remember to color your set up phrases with all the negative, ugly, hurtful thoughts that you hear in your head when you look at your body. Keep tapping until you feel relaxed and you feel the intensity subside. Then finish up with a positive affirmation:

Even though my body isn't perfect, it is my body temple, and it supports my life, and I choose to deeply and completely love and accept all of myself.

Body Beliefs

Now that you've done your body inventory, next we'll do some more tapping for the negative feelings and limiting beliefs we have surrounding our bodies. You can formulate your own personal set up phrases by filling in the blanks provided:

Even though my body is so _____, I choose to deeply and completely love and accept myself.

Even though I can't stand looking at my _____

Even though my thighs are _____

Even though my butt looks _____

Even though no one will want to have sex with me because _____

Even though seeing my naked body in the mirror makes me feel
_____,

Even though I feel inadequate, and my body's not enough

Even though I hate my body

Even though I'm as big as a house

Even though I feel like an elephant

Even though I can't stand looking in the mirror

Even though I feel fat, and always have

Even though I believe I'm ugly

Even though I'm ashamed of my body

Even though I refuse to accept my body as it is

Even though I feel huge and fat when I look at myself

Even though I have cottage cheese thighs

Even though I have a jiggly buddha belly

Even though _____ shamed me about my body

Even though I'm mad at him/her for saying _____

Even though he/she hurt my self-esteem

Even though I felt hurt, and thought I would never be good enough

Even though I started to believe I was fat because of what he/she/they said

Even though I felt so judged by what he/she/they said

Even though I'm afraid of intimacy because I'll be rejected

Now finish up with,

Even though I can't accept my body the way it is now, I now choose to deeply and completely accept all of myself ANYWAY.

EB	I want to learn how to love my body
SE	I want to learn how to feel comfortable with my body
UE	I would like to enjoy how my body looks
UN	I choose to learn how to love my body
CH	I choose to learn to accept my body
CB	I choose to approve of my body and myself
UA	I want to learn how to love myself
TH	I choose to learn to love ALL of me

Be sure to tap in several rounds of the above to affirm acceptance and appreciation for your body and all it does for you each and every day. Think of the thousands of heartbeats, breaths you take, and all the other cellular activity your body does each day all on its own. Your body works very hard, and should be acknowledged, appreciated and loved. It is a gift from God. It houses your very soul!

Body Pain

Another body related issue is body pain. I've noticed in my practice that some of my clients with food addictions also suffer from chronic pain or other ailments which sap their energy, vitality and general sense of joy in life. It's not uncommon for overweight people to have problems with things like joint or back pain. Dealing with any kind of body pain day in and day out is exhausting and can cause a great deal of anger and sadness. There may also be a sense of giving up on life, a loss of hope. These feelings can cause us to turn to food as the only source of comfort in our lives. We feel like we can forget our pain momentarily if we can just have a sweet dessert or our favorite snack.

Do you suffer from chronic pain? If you do, close your eyes and take a moment to examine this pain. Where is your pain located within your body? What are the qualities of your pain? Can you describe the size, shape and feeling of your pain? Is it sharp, burning hot, and localized? Is it like a knife stabbing you? Or is it a continuous dull ache?

———————————————————————————————

———————————————————————————————

———————————————————————————————

———————————————————————————————

How does having this chronic pain make you feel?

_____

_____

_____

_____

Now tap for all your thoughts about how your pain limits you and makes you sad or angry. You can use the sample set ups below by adding in your own personal details. Tap until you feel that all your sadness and anger has been released.

Even though I have this _____ pain, I deeply and completely love and accept myself.

Even though I have this chronic _____ pain

Even though this pain makes me feel _____

Even though I feel enraged by my pain

Even though I feel resentful that I can't live a normal life

Even though my pain limits me and makes me feel hopeless and helpless

Even though I'm angry that no one understands how hard it is for me

Even though I have this anger and resentment, I choose to love and accept myself anyway

Even though this is a physical problem and I don't think EFT will help for it

Even though I don't deserve to get better

Even though I have this dull ache

Even though it feels like a knife is twisting in my

Even though I have this shooting pain

Even though I have this searing pain

Even though I have this burning pain

Even though I have this excruciating pain and all the emotional hurt that is causing it

Even though I have this tightness in my _____

Even though I have this ache in my _____

Even though I have this pain when I try to _____

Even though I'm angry that I've had to go through so much

Even though I'm enraged that I have to suffer with this chronic pain

Even though I have this anger and resentment in my (body part)

Even though I have this sadness in my (body part)

Even though this pain prevents me from having a normal life

Even though I have this pain in the butt/ pain in the neck/ pain in my _____

Even though I have this _____ pain, I choose to deeply and completely love and accept myself anyway.

Fibromyalgia and Chronic Pain

Interestingly, I've found that many food addicts frequently also suffer from arthritis, or other chronic inflammatory pain of some sort. It has been my experience that chronic pain is the body's way of expressing emotional and spiritual pain that has been suppressed for many years. It's our body's way of calling attention to something that needs to be dealt with in order for us to truly experience health, happiness and inner peace. Many chronic pain sufferers have a tendency to hold back their self-expression and not say what they really feel. As children we are keenly aware of whatever it is we have to do to earn our parents' love and affection. This could mean having to perform, but it could just as easily mean suppressing our real thoughts and feelings if they conflict with those of our parents. This sets up a pattern of pushing our needs and desires down and holding ourselves back. The years of repressing the self, and the negative thoughts, beliefs and emotions that accompany it ultimately results in anger, rage, sadness and grief that demand expression.

Fibromyalgia is another ailment that is not uncommon among food addicts. Although the exact mechanism that causes fibromyalgia has not been identified, some experts hypothesize that the central nervous system of fibromyalgia sufferers differs from that of a normal person in that it is overly active, or more "sensitive". Chronic pain is viewed as a disturbance in a sensitive person's electrical system triggered by an emotional trauma of some sort. Fortunately, Dr. Joaquin Andrade showed us that EFT has the effect of re-organizing the brain and calming the nervous system. This may be in part why EFT has proven to be so effective in relieving fibromyalgia and other chronic pain.

Most people are taught to believe that pain is a real, physical condition that has no emotional component whatsoever and is therefore set in stone. But John Sarno, MD, author of "Mind Over Back Pain", disagrees. Dr. Sarno found that chronic pain has a psychological component. As a practicing physician, Dr. Sarno began to notice a difference in patients' back x-rays. He observed that some patients with obvious spine abnormalities experienced no pain, while other patients with no observable spine abnormalities suffered from chronic pain. This led him to study the phenomenon and develop his theory of TMS or Tension Myositis Syndrome. Dr. Sarno theorizes that TMS is a syndrome whereby suppressed rage and anxiety causes pain by restricting blood flow to tissues. While his theory is not fully embraced by the mainstream medical establishment, Dr. Sarno claims to obtain good results when he treats patients for their underlying emotional distress.

If you, too, believe that certain ailments are organic, or that genetics determine what you will and won't experience in your body, I would invite you re-examine the idea of what "genetic" actually means and check out the latest research in the field of epigenetics. You may begin to doubt that there is such a thing as a "genetic" condition at all. Epigenetics is the study of how gene expression is affected by influences other than changes in gene DNA.

As it turns out, many things can influence if and how a gene is expressed in the human body. Scientists observed that all organisms with the same genotype (genetic makeup) do not necessarily display the same phenotype (the observable traits and physical characteristics of an organism). This led to the study of epigenetics, or the study of any outside influence which moderates gene expression. Such influences include, but aren't limited to, emotions and environmental stress.

Do you suffer from chronic pain or fibromyalgia? Has anyone ever told you that you're "too sensitive"? Do you take things very personally? Can you feel the energy in a room? Are you sensitive to other people's emotions? Do loud noises bother you? Do crowded, noisy places overload your circuits? In all probability you might be what is called a clinically "sensitive" person. There is a specific personality type that has been identified by Elaine Aron called a Highly Sensitive Person. On the Kiersey Bates psychological temperament scale, you would be considered an "intuitive feeler" (an NF type).

Does any of this sound familiar? If so, you are probably a highly sensitive person too, and as such you're much more prone to emotional assaults and hurt feelings. Sensitive types have a more delicate nervous system and are also more susceptible to stress, and more sensitive to traumatic events. But that's okay. Being a sensitive person puts you more in touch with your spiritual nature. It also makes you a creator of beauty and a bringer of light to the world. We simply need to honor our sensitivity, and tap to release the hurts we have already experienced in our lives so we can be set free.

Another way of looking at chronic pain is to examine the secondary benefits we derive from it. It may sound crazy to say that we get any benefits from chronic pain, but if we really take the time to examine it a little deeper, we may see what function pain actually serves in our life.

Audrey was the wife of a prominent political figure in her city. We discussed her fibromyalgia and how it might actually have a subconscious message for her. I asked her what her life would be like without the pain. She took a second to respond and said to her own amazement, "Ugh, I would have to go to all those functions. I would have to play the role of the Mayor's wife. Having fibromyalgia gives me a legitimate excuse to get out of going. It gives me the right to say no to anything I don't really want to do. It gives me the power to say NO!"

Chronic pain usually serves the purpose of allowing us to say no to someone or something in our lives - like a job we hate, or a demanding spouse or family member. I believe that a good many folks currently on disability have found a way to say no to a disappointing job, or life, in a way that is socially acceptable. I believe that if they were able to deal with the sadness and disappointment inside, they might be able to not only finally be well, but also create a life that they really enjoyed living – free of pain.

If you suffer from chronic pain, I invite you to examine what purpose your fibromyalgia/chronic pain might serve in your life.

Ask yourself:

If your body pain had a message for you, what would it be?

_____

_____

_____

_____

Does it allow you to say "no" to anyone or anything, without feeling guilty? If so, to what or whom?

_____

_____

_____

_____

Does it give you control over who has access to you and when?

_____

_____

_____

_____

Does it allow you to establish boundaries that you don't feel comfortable setting otherwise? To say no to favors, activities, or chores you don't really want to do? Which ones?

_____

_____

_____

_____

Does it enable you to have some "me" time doing things that you want to do, instead of what others want you to do? Does it give you time to sleep, watch TV, read or do crafts?

_____

_____

_____

_____

_____

Does it enable you to be waited on by family members? Does it gain you attention or pampering you feel you wouldn't otherwise receive?

_____

_____

_____

_____

_____

_____

Tap on all your insights resulting from your answers to the above questions, and then see if you identify with any of the sample set ups below.

Even though I feel very sad and depressed about my pain

Even though I'm angry and sad that my body hurts all over

Even though I am so disappointed in my life

Even though it doesn't feel safe to express myself

Even though it was never safe to say what I really wanted or really felt growing up

Even though my unexpressed thoughts and emotions are manifesting as pain

Even though this is my way of being heard

Even though I don't honor my own needs as being important

Even though I take care of everyone else first instead of me

Even though I'm overwhelmed with all of the things that are going on in my life

Even though loud, crowded places bother me

Even though I'm overly sensitive to noise

Even though I take a lot of things people do and say personally

Even though I'm easily hurt, sad and depressed

Even though if I get well people might expect too much of me

Even though if I get better I might expect too much of myself

Even though having chronic pain/fibromyalgia lets me control how much I have to do, when and for whom

Even though having this pain gives me the power to say "no"

Even though this pain gets me attention and pampering

Even though I need to keep this pain so I don't have to go to work

Even though I'm afraid I'll have to go back to work if I get better

EB   I choose to see that I can get better
SE   I choose to realize that it's safe for me to get well
UE   I see now that I can safely express myself and my needs
UN   I choose to see it's safe to reclaim my power
CH   I choose to believe it's possible to live a happy, healthy life
CB   I choose to be open to the idea of fulfilling my dreams
UA   I choose to be happy and take care of my own needs
TH   I choose to deeply and profoundly love, accept and cherish myself

Whether you realize it or not, by this point in the book, you've come the majority of the way on your journey toward eliminating your food addiction problem. You've unearthed and released many deeply buried emotions including sadness, anxiety, anger, guilt, shame, as well as heavy personal traumas. These are the emotions which were the driving force behind your compulsive eating behavior. The only things which could prevent your further progress are your own limiting beliefs and self-sabotaging behavior. We'll be dealing with those issues in the next chapter.

Chapter 8

Self-Sabotage

As food addicts, we face certain challenges when trying to lose weight. In addition to the emotions that compel us to overeat, we very often harbor beliefs that sabotage our efforts at weight loss. We can't expect to make any real progress in our weight loss efforts until all our resistance to losing the weight has been eliminated. This chapter is devoted to helping you weed out your self-sabotaging beliefs and emotions. Really spend some time reflecting on your answers to the questions in this chapter, because those answers are the key to finally allowing yourself to lose the weight once and for all.

Secondary Gains

As I mentioned in the previous chapter, secondary gains are the benefits that we receive from hanging onto a problem. I think very few people would consciously choose to be in pain. But with food addiction, it's very probable that our compulsive eating behavior and overweight are filling a vital, protective role in our lives. It's very likely that our favorite foods are comforting us, nurturing us, and protecting us in a way we desperately need. So even though we may consciously want to lose the extra weight and stop overeating, our subconscious mind rebels against that idea. Part of us wants to lose the weight, while another part of us needs everything to stay the same. So what ends up happening is that we engage in self-sabotage to make sure no one takes away our beloved food. Ask yourself:

Why do you think you are sabotaging your weight loss efforts?

_____

_____

_____

_____

_____

Do you think there are any positive aspects to keeping your weight? What is the upside to remaining overweight?

_____

_____

_____

_____

What are the possible downsides to losing the weight?

_____

_____

_____

_____

_____

Were you surprised at all by your answers? Take a moment to create set up phrases for each one of the insights you gained and tap for each one.

In the following sections, we'll be addressing common stumbling blocks faced by food addicts when attempting to lose weight.

It's Not Safe to Lose the Weight

Most food addicts tend to fail in their weight loss efforts because subconsciously it feels safer to remain the way they are, rather than lose the weight. Sometimes it's easier to live the limited life we're familiar with, than try and change for the better. Change can be very scary. It's much easier to stick with the life we know, than to face the unknown. Can you think of any reasons why you might not want to lose the weight? To see if fear might be holding you back, try answering the following questions:

Is it really safe for you to lose the overweight? In what way could losing the weight be unsafe or threatening? What's the worst thing that could happen if you lost the weight?

_____

What in your life will have to change or be different if you lose the weight? What will happen when you become thin?

Now take each one of the answers to the previous questions and turn them into as many set up phrases as you can. Tap on each one of them. When you're finished, review the sample set ups below and tap on them too, adding your own words and phrasing as you desire.

KC   Even though I'm afraid to lose the weight, I deeply and completely love and accept myself.

KC   Even though it's not safe for me to lose weight, I deeply and profoundly love and accept myself.

KC   Even though I'm afraid I won't feel safe without my food, I choose to deeply and completely love and accept myself anyway.

EB	Even though it's not safe for me to lose weight
SE	Even though I'm afraid to change
UE	I'm afraid to leave my comfort zone
UN	I don't feel safe letting go of my food
CH	I feel scared about getting thinner
CB	I'm afraid I won't feel safe anymore without my shield
UA	Even though I feel unsafe about getting thinner
TH	I'm afraid to lose weight because I don't know who I would be

EB	The thought of losing weight makes me feel threatened
SE	And I'm afraid to feel vulnerable again
UE	Even though I can't protect myself without the weight
UN	Even though I feel safer with protection
CH	Even though I'd be forced to change and I'd be afraid
CB	I can feel safe about changing my life for the better
UA	I choose to feel safe about losing the weight
TH	I now choose to feel safe, happy and peaceful about losing the weight once and for all

EB	Even though it's not safe for me to lose the weight
SE	Even though it's not safe for me to achieve my goal
UE	I don't know why I have this resistance
UN	And I've been sabotaging my progress so I don't have to change
CH	So I can stay where I am, where I'm more comfortable
CB	With this weight I know who I am
UA	I don't know who I would I be if I changed and lost the weight
TH	I now choose to feel peaceful about losing the weight

EB   What if losing the weight doesn't solve all my problems
SE   What if I lose the weight and I still hate my life
UE   What if it doesn't work, and I'm still unhappy
UN   I now choose to feel safe about losing weight
CH   I choose to feel hopeful and positive about losing the weight
CB   I am willing to realize that I have the power to change
UA   I choose to understand that I can be successful
TH   I choose to believe that is safe and easy to lose the weight

Reactions from Others

Sometimes we're afraid of other people's possible reactions to our weight loss. We're afraid we'll lose our connections to family members or close friends. We're afraid of losing our closest relationships, or that our loved ones will become jealous or envious of us. It's important to work through these powerfully limiting beliefs so we can achieve our weight loss goals.

Ask yourself:

Would someone be threatened by your weight loss? How will the other people in your life respond to you if you lose the weight? Will they be envious, jealous, angry or become aloof? Will your family stop loving you? Could your friends dump you?

_____

_____

_____

_____

_____

What are your beliefs about thin people? Do you think they are conceited, or snobby or "fake"? Do you believe people will think that way about you if you lose the weight?

_____

_____

_____

_____

_____

Have you lost a large amount of weight before? If so, what happened the last time you were at your goal weight? Did something happen to cause you not to want to lose weight again?

_____

_____

_____

_____

Turn each answer above into as many set up phrases as you can think of, and tap on them. When you're done, tap on the set up phrases below.

KC   Even though it's not safe for others if I lose weight, I deeply and completely love and accept myself.

KC   Even though they won't understand if I lose the weight, I choose to love and accept all of me.

KC   Even though I'm afraid of what they'll think if I lose the weight, I choose to deeply and profoundly love and accept myself.

EB   Even though I'm afraid they will _____
SE   And I'm afraid they'll say _____
UE   I'm afraid they'll reject me
UN   I'm afraid they'll stop loving me
CH   Even though some people might stop giving me attention
CB   I can choose to feel safe about losing the weight
UA   I choose to feel confident, and loved and supported
TH   I choose to be happy and hopeful about my weight loss

KC   Even though I'll feel guilty for losing weight and being thinner than _____ (my mother / sister / friend), I deeply and completely love and accept myself.

KC   Even though I'm sabotaging my diet to protect _____ (my mother/ sister/ friend), I deeply and profoundly love and accept myself.

KC   Even though I can't be successful without _____ (my mother's / sister's/ friend's) support, I choose to deeply and completely love and accept myself anyway.

EB   Even though I'm afraid he/she might feel _____ if I lost the weight
SE   And I'm afraid of being disloyal to _____
UE   And I don't want _____ to be envious of me
UN   I don't want _____ to be jealous of me
CH   I don't want people to think I'm _____
CB   I don't want _____ to reject me
UA   I choose to feel loved and accepted in my life
TH   I choose to feel comfortable losing the weight

EB   Even though _____ won't give me his/her support if I'm successful
SE   And I don't feel supported by my family members in my weight loss
UE   Even though they always try to sabotage me with food to make me stay fat
UN   Even though I sabotage myself to stay fat
CH   I choose to feel loved and supported
CB   I choose to feel accepted
UA   I choose to love and support myself
TH   I choose to feel loved and supported in my life

KC   Even though I might receive unwanted attention if I become thin, I deeply and completely love and accept myself.

KC   Even though I might get unwanted attention if I become slender, I choose to love and accept myself anyway.

KC   Even though some people might stare at me, I choose to feel safe, and confident and powerful.

EB   What if I get more attention than I really want
SE   What if I get attention I don't want
UE   What if people stare at me
UN   People will look at me differently
CH   People will judge me
CB   What if people still don't like me after I lose the weight
UA   What if I don't have any more friends when I lose the weight
TH   What if I lose the weight and no one is attracted to me after all

EB   I choose to see it differently now
SE   I choose to understand I can be safe at my goal weight
UE   I am willing to learn to enjoy being thin
UN   I want to learn how to be thin and confident
CH   I want to learn how to be healthy and strong
CB   I choose to feel confident and accepted
UA   I choose to accept my body completely
TH   I choose to feel peaceful about being slender

It's Just Too Hard

Sometimes the thought of all the weight we have to lose is very daunting. We feel that it's just too hard, or too much effort. We doubt our abilities not only to lose the weight, but to keep it off.

210

We're going to tap now for these feelings of being overwhelmed. Start by asking yourself:

Do you believe you can't lose the weight? Why can't you?

_____

_____

_____

_____

Do you doubt your ability to keep the weight off? Why?

_____

_____

_____

_____

After tapping for your answers above, tap on the set ups below:

KC   Even though I feel losing the weight is just too hard, I deeply and completely love and accept myself.

KC   Even though I feel discouraged by how much weight I have to lose, I completely accept my feelings and emotions.

KC   Even though I feel angry and overwhelmed that I have all this weight to lose, I choose to accept myself and my emotions now.

EB   Even though I'm mad at myself because I have to go through this again

SE   And I'm frustrated that I gained all this weight

UE   Even though my weight loss goes way too slow

UN   Even though I can't eat like other people

CH   Even though I have to exercise every day in order to lose weight

CB   Even though my body doesn't want to let go of the weight

UA   Even though my body refuses to let go of the weight

TH   I choose to believe that it can be easy for me to lose weight

EB   I don't think I can lose the weight permanently

SE   I'll probably gain it all back anyway

UE   What if I gain the weight back

UN   I probably will

CH   I'll probably gain back all the weight like I always have

CB   And it always has to be a struggle to keep the weight off

UA   Even though I will continually have to deprive myself in order to keep the weight off

TH   And I'll constantly have to be on guard or else I'll gain it right back again

EB   Because I've always been fat
SE   I'll always be fat
UE   I wish I could lose the weight once and for all
UN   I really want to lose the weight and be healthy
CH   I know I can lose the weight
CB   I've done it before
UA   I choose to feel relaxed and peaceful about losing weight
TH   I choose to feel easy and confident about losing the weight

EB   I choose to live a healthier lifestyle
SE   I choose to soothe myself in healthier ways than junk food
UE   I choose to make healthy choices
UN   I choose to make healthier decisions
CH   I choose to enjoy my life right now
CB   I choose to embrace health now
UA   I choose to love and support myself now
TH   I choose to feel easy and calm about losing the weight

I'm A Failure: I Don't Deserve to Lose the Weight

One extraordinarily sabotaging belief we can hold is that we are a failure. It makes us doubt our ability to accomplish the goals we set in our lives, including weight loss. It's imperative that we banish this belief so we can reach our weight loss goals. Here are some set ups that can help do this:

KC   Even though I'm not sure if I'm worthy of succeeding, I choose to deeply and completely accept myself.

KC Even though I don't feel like I deserve to be thin, I deeply and completely love and accept myself.

KC Even though I'm a failure and I don't deserve to be thin, I choose to feel worthy and accepted now.

EB Even though I don't deserve to achieve my goal
SE I don't deserve to be happy with my body
UE Even though I fail at everything I try and do
UN Even though I have no reason to believe I'll be successful at losing the weight this time
CH Even though I don't feel like I can achieve my goal
CB Even though I'm a loser and always have been a loser
UA Because I'm only a dreamer who never follows through on anything
TH I don't know even how to be successful at losing weight

EB Even though I'm never successful at what I want to do
SE Even though I don't feel safe when I'm successful
UE I choose to believe I can be successful
UN I choose to feel safe being successful
CH I choose to know that I can do it
CB I choose to lose the weight now
UA I choose to live a healthy lifestyle
TH I choose to enjoy my life right now

Getting In Your Own Way: Fear of Success

Sometimes we have trouble picturing our life as a thin person. Being thin seems outside our realm of experience. To find out if you have some subconscious resistance to losing weight, here's an exercise for you to try. While sitting in a comfortable chair, close your eyes and take a few deep breaths. Now imagine yourself at your goal weight. Are you having trouble picturing it? That's okay. Just relax and try to imagine what your daily life would be like IF you were at your goal weight. Make the picture as clear and vivid as you possibly can. Try and feel the emotions you would feel as a thin person. Imagine how your body feels. Imagine what you would do on a daily basis. Where would you go? How would people react to you in your new body? What thoughts rush into your mind when you think about this?

What negative feelings came up for you as you did this? When you imagined yourself at your goal weight, did any "yeah buts..." come up. In EFT we call those "tail enders", and they need to be addressed in order to make full progress toward change. Tail enders are negative beliefs that stand between us and our truest desires.

List any negative reactions, or "yeah buts" you experienced during your visualization here:

_____

_____

_____

_____

_____

_____

What were some of the negative feelings you felt or what resistance did you feel when you tried to imagine yourself as slender?

_____

_____

_____

_____

Be sure to tap on each one of the "yeah buts" you identified from answering those questions. When you feel you're done, read and tap along with the sample set ups below:

KC   Even though I have a block of some sort to weighing _____ pounds (your goal weight), I deeply and completely love and accept myself.

KC   Even though I try and sabotage myself whenever I reach my goal weight, I deeply and profoundly accept myself.

KC   Even though I'm using my weight as a way to get in my own way, and hold myself back, I choose to deeply and completely love and accept anyway.

EB	Even though I can't picture myself reaching my goal
SE	And I'm having difficulty seeing myself at my goal weight
UE	And I've been sabotaging my progress
UN	Because I don't know how to be a success at losing weight
CH	And I've been holding on to these blocks for so long
CB	Now I choose to release those blocks
UA	I choose to feel comfortable releasing my blocks to losing weight
TH	I choose to believe I can reach my goal weight

EB	Even though I don't feel comfortable losing the weight again
SE	And I don't feel safe leaving my comfort zone
UE	I'm more comfortable staying overweight
UN	Because with this weight I know who I am
CH	I don't know what I would really be like if I changed and lost the weight
CB	What if I lose the weight and become saggy and wrinkly
UA	I'm afraid of looking old and wrinkly
TH	I choose to feel safe and comfortable losing the weight

EB	I want to feel safe
SE	I want to feel healthy and happy
UE	I want to allow myself to lose the weight
UN	I choose to allow myself to feel safe and comfortable losing the weight
CH	I choose to allow myself to be happy and peaceful
CB	I choose to allow myself to give up the weight
UA	I choose to stop carrying around my excess weight
TH	I choose to finally let go and release the weight

Here are some questions to stimulate your thoughts about your attitudes toward success:

What are some of the other obstacles that you currently experience to successfully losing weight? Are there any behaviors you engage in that sabotage your efforts? Do you have any theories as to why you do these behaviors?

_____

_____

_____

_____

_____

What sort of negative self-talk goes on in your head when you think about dieting or losing weight? Some of the negative things I tell myself are:

_____

_____

_____

_____

If I had to guess why I think and do these things to sabotage my weight loss success, I would say:

_____

_____

_____

_____

Did you see a pattern of fear of success in your answers? Go ahead and tap for all the insights that came out of answering those questions. Here are some other common set ups relating to fear of success that I often hear from my food addiction clients:

KC   Even though success does not feel safe, I deeply and completely love and accept myself.

KC   Even though I'm sabotaging my weight loss to protect myself, I deeply and profoundly love and accept myself.

KC   Even though success does not feel good, I choose to deeply and completely love and accept myself anyway.

EB   Even though I'm afraid to be a big success
SE   Even though success feels threatening
UE   Part of me doesn't want to succeed
UN   Part of me doesn't want to change
CH   I'm not allowed to be a success
CB   It just doesn't feel right

UA   I choose to accept that I can be a success

TH   I choose to understand that I can be comfortable being a success

KC   Even though maybe I don't really want to get over this food addiction, I deeply and completely love and accept myself.

KC   Even though I might not really want to be healed of my compulsive eating, I deeply and profoundly love and accept myself.

KC   Even though I might not want to be a normal, healthy weight person, I choose to love and accept myself anyway.

EB   Even though it may not be safe to give up my food addiction

SE   I might not even know how to act if I didn't have this food addiction

UE   I am willing to feel safe about giving up my food addiction

UN   I choose to feel safe about losing the weight

CH   I choose to feel good about my weight loss success

CB   I choose to feel positive and expectant about losing weight

UA   I am willing to believe I can be successful

TH   I choose to know it's possible for me to be successful

KC   Even though being successful might mean more responsibility, I deeply and completely love and accept myself.

KC   Even though I'm afraid that people will expect more of me if I lose weight and become successful, I deeply and profoundly love and accept myself.

KC   Even though it might mean I'll have to KEEP being successful, and I don't think I can do it, I choose to relax and completely love and accept myself anyway.

EB   Even though more may be required of me if I lose the weight
SE   And I'll be expected to achieve if I lose the weight
UE   I'll be expected to perform
UN   I'll have to do more
CH   Even though I've always been an underachiever
CB   Even though it feels comfortable and familiar to be unhappy
UA   Even though I've never been successful, and I don't know how to be
TH   I'm willing to accept the possibility that I can be successful

EB   Even though I'll need to work hard
SE   Even though I don't think I can ever achieve my goal
UE   If I were to achieve my goals, I might be forced to change
UN   I don't know why I have this resistance to changing and becoming successful
CH   Even though change feels so overwhelming
CB   Success feels overwhelming

UA   Being a success feels frightening and different
TH   I choose to believe it is safe to change a become a success

EB   But what if I lose the weight and people still don't like me
SE   What if I'm successful and they still don't like me
UE   What if I'm successful and people find out I'm a fraud
UN   Everyone will know I'm a fraud
CH   Because I know I'm a fraud
CB   What if I believed I could be successful
UA   I choose to believe I can be successful now
TH   I choose to believe it is safe for me to be a success

EB   Even though being a success means I'll lose my support
SE   I'm afraid of feeling alone and unsupported
UE   I am afraid I'll be lonely
UN   Even though I'm afraid I won't be cared for anymore if I'm successful
CH   My parents will no longer help me
CB   Even though it is safer not to even try
UA   I choose to feel loved and supported anyway
TH   I choose to feel safe about my weight loss and success

KC   Even though I can't be successful without _____'s support, I deeply and completely love and accept myself.

KC   Even though he/she won't give me his/her support if I'm successful, I deeply and profoundly love and accept myself anyway.

KC Even though if I lost weight then I'd be free of _____ and I wouldn't know what to do, I choose to love and accept myself and my feelings.

EB I'm afraid I'd have to live my own life for myself and not for others
SE And I wouldn't know how to be in the world
UE Even though I'm afraid of success if I lose weight
UN I choose to feel confident and peaceful
CH I choose to own my power and be successful
CB I choose to forge my own way
UA I choose to create a life of happiness
TH I choose to be peaceful and happy about my success

Now that you've completed tapping for anything that you feel might be sabotaging your weight loss efforts, we're going to finish up with tapping in a few rounds of positive affirmations.

🦋 Exercise: Tapping on Affirmations

Throughout the book you've been alternately tapping on negative reminder phrases and positive statements during the tapping rounds. Tapping on positive statements helps reinforce the gains you made while tapping on a particular set up phrase, as well as permanently anchor a positive reframe to your negative thoughts and beliefs. But tapping on a positive statement can also be used as kind of a high-octane affirmation. Many times when we recite positive affirmations to ourselves, we meet with internal resistance because we don't feel like the statement is true for us. Anyone who has repeated the affirmation "I am a millionaire" immediately feels that the statement is not empirically true for them at the moment.

But there's a way that we can make an affirmation much more agreeable, powerful, and therefore more likely to manifest in our lives. If we simply add the words, "I choose to" or "I now choose to", it becomes something we can really get on board with. After all, who wouldn't choose to be a millionaire, or choose to be happy, or choose to be fulfilled? We're very comfortable with making choices. We make hundreds of them every day.

In this exercise, you'll be crafting 5 personal affirmations that you'll tap on each day, in the morning and evening. You can also tap on them whenever you have any down time, like in the car, in the shower or even during commercials. You simply tap on the 8 tapping points and omit the karate chop point. The affirmations should reflect your deepest intentions for overcoming your food addiction and your hopes for your future, like so:

I choose to love, honor and accept myself, regardless of my weight.

I choose to live a life of peace, freedom and fulfillment.

I choose to feel loved, loving, and lovable at all times.

I now choose to honor and nourish my body with healthy foods.

I now choose to feel worthy of all good things coming into my life.

I now choose to accept my success.

I now choose to believe I deserve success.

I choose to allow my success now.

I now choose to begin enjoying my success.

I now choose to live a fulfilling life of happiness, purpose and abundance.

As you design your affirmations, think about the way you would like to feel, and the way you would like your life to be in the future. It may be helpful to look back over your set up phrases from earlier in the chapter and write a choice that is exactly the opposite of one of them. Write your personal affirmation choices in the spaces provided:

I (now) choose to_____.

I (now) choose to_____.

I (now) choose to_____.

I (now) choose to_____.

I (now) choose to_____.

Once you've created your choice affirmations, transcribe them onto 3 x 5 cards and keep them with you to refer to periodically, or put them on your night table so you can review them in the morning and the evening. Feel free to write more than 5 if you feel inspired to do so. You can never have too much positive affirmation in your life!

Chapter 9

The Fire Within: Your Metabolism

A lifetime of chronic yo-yo dieting combined with binge eating can take its toll on our metabolism. This can make weight loss very frustrating, as our metabolism seems to have shut down and our body appears to be betraying us. Our poor body expects to be starved again at any moment and our endocrine system reacts by causing us to retain calories. What ends up happening is that ultimately our metabolism becomes so slow that we require very few calories to live, and thus very few more calories to gain weight and build up fat. On top of that, the carbohydrate-laden foods we eat, like sweets and starches, create a huge surge of insulin – a hormone that can wreak havoc in our bodies if it remains at chronically high levels. Not only do high insulin levels contribute to heart disease, they can make weight loss nearly impossible.

As a side note, menopause can be an extremely difficult time to attempt to lose weight. I experienced my own challenges in this area due to a hysterectomy. I recommend that menopausal women find a knowledgeable doctor who can discuss bio-identical hormone replacement options and evaluate your thyroid function. Estrogen dominance syndrome can mimic thyroid dysfunction and adding some bio-identical progesterone cream can often help, as was the case for me. Hormone imbalance can cause insulin resistance, weight gain, and persistent hunger. I recommend Dr. John R. Lee and Virginia Hopkins' books, "What Your Doctor May Not Tell You About Menopause" and "Hormone Balance Made Simple" for any woman going through menopause. The information they contain is invaluable in my opinion.

I also encourage everyone who wishes to lose weight to try and eat unprocessed, protein rich foods, as well as more natural foods like fruits, vegetables and nuts. As a former carbohydrate addict, I noticed that the more high-carb, sugary foods I ate, the more I wanted. Eating carbs was a trigger for me to eat even more carbs. I never experienced this kind of compulsion when I ate fruits and vegetables, only cookies, pasta and bread. Now I personally try not to eat anything that comes in a box or can, as it is likely to be highly processed, and contain large amounts of preservatives, sugar, salt, or MSG. I realize that it may not be possible to completely eliminate these foods at the start. But if you begin to cut down, while incorporating more raw, organic and unprocessed foods into your diet, your body will respond with increased energy, vitality and health. Eating predominantly in this manner still allows you to occasionally enjoy things that aren't as good for you, like a plate of pasta, dessert or café mocha. If you're feeding your body mostly fresh, organic and healthy foods, it will be more forgiving when you do occasionally indulge.

Emotions And Your Metabolism

Chances are after years of dieting, your metabolism could use a little kick start. EFT has been shown to be surprisingly effective for thyroid and other metabolism issues. Your body's metabolism is governed primarily by the glands of the endocrine system, and these glands are greatly impacted by negative emotions of all kinds including anger, grief, sadness, and disappointment. And since EFT is able to dissolve these negative emotions very efficiently, it is able to clear the way for the endocrine system to

228

begin functioning normally. However, I want to stress here that you should never go off any of your medications, including thyroid medication, without first obtaining the approval of your doctor.

In Louise Hay's famous book, "You can Heal Your Life" she associates thyroid problems with the emotional themes of "not getting to do what you want to do", stifled creative expression, and limitation. But other emotions can affect the thyroid and other endocrine glands as well, like depression, anger or hopelessness. That's why it's so important to tap when we feel a negative emotion coming on, or have an insight about what may be causing our fear, anger or sadness.

Amy came to see me for her food addiction. She had been on many diets, and had great difficulty losing weight. She was also very tired, depressed and felt achy all over. She was contemplating making an appointment to see her doctor for blood tests and to possibly go on thyroid medication. As we discussed her childhood, Amy revealed how her mother had been very angry, controlling and punitive towards her. Amy felt like she could never say what she wanted or "talk back" to her mother, because it would cause her to fly into a rage. Challenging her mother would only lead to yelling and spankings, followed by being ignored by her mother until Amy finally apologized to her mother for whatever transgression she committed. This dynamic with her mother taught Amy that she "had no say", and that her wants and opinions didn't matter.

The thyroid gland is often associated with creative expression or giving voice to one's wants and desires. I felt Amy needed to "find her voice". So I had her tap on "Even though I could never have what I wanted", "Even though mom got furious whenever I

229

disagreed with her", "Even though I was always punished for talking back", "Even though I was ignored whenever she got angry", "Even though I learned that my needs don't count", and "Even though I never had a right to my own voice and opinions, I now choose to express myself with confidence. I choose to have my say. I have a right to my own opinions." After our session, Amy said she felt much lighter and was glad that she made the connection between finding her voice and her thyroid issues. When I spoke to her after our meeting, Amy was enjoying more energy and said her body aches were gone, and she was no longer binge eating.

If you have thyroid or other metabolic issues, I would encourage you to take a look at where you might be suppressing your voice, your wants and desires. Think about whether you have difficulties saying no to anyone, or whether you try and please people by doing what they want, instead of what you want. If you identify with some of these issues, you may want to tap for the following set ups:

Even though I could never have what I wanted

Even though it wasn't safe for me to express myself, or I would be punished

Even though I was taught that I have no right to my own thoughts and opinions

Even though I was taught that my opinions don't matter

Even though I learned that my needs don't count

Even though I learned that I was wrong

Even though I learned that I shouldn't want what I want

Even though I could never say NO to my mother/father /_____or I would get spanked/beaten/ _____

Even though expressing myself got me into trouble, so I just shut down

Even though I stopped expressing myself to avoid the pain, I choose to see that I have a right to my own voice.

Even though it's just easier to go along with what others want, I now choose to see that it's okay to express myself easily and confidently. I choose to accept my own power with ease and love.

Metabolic Kick Start

We can also tap for our metabolic processes directly, and to speed up our metabolism and balance our hormones. So, in order to give our body a little kick start, we're going to tap for an increased metabolism. Tap along with the following set ups:

KC   Even though my metabolism is too slow, I deeply and completely love and accept myself.

KC   Even though my metabolism is imbalanced, I deeply and completely love and accept myself.

KC   Even though I'm frustrated with my body for being so sluggish, I choose to deeply and completely accept all of me, even my body.

EB   Even though everyone in my family is overweight
SE   And I can't fight my genes
UE   Even though my body is too old to change now
UN   Even though my metabolism died after my 20's/30's
CH   Even though my metabolism decreased after I had my kids
CB   Even though my metabolism shut down after menopause
UA   And people always gain weight as they get older
TH   I choose to allow myself to have a faster metabolism

EB   Even though my body is betraying me
SE   Even though my body wants to hold on to the weight and not let go
UE   And I can't seem to eat as much as other people can without gaining weight
UN   And I can't seem to overcome my sluggish metabolism
CH   Even though I have a slower metabolism than other people
CB   Even though my hormones are out of balance
UA   Even though my body is out of balance
TH   I now choose to have a faster, healthier metabolism

EB   I now choose to have a faster metabolism
SE   I allow my endocrine system to function perfectly
UE   I allow my thyroid and other glands to work perfectly
UN   All my glands and my organs work together in harmony
CH   I'm ready to release this weight and become balanced again

CB   I now ask my body to return to perfect balance
UA   I ask my metabolism to speed up
TH   I ask my body to increase my metabolism

Increasing Your Metabolism: Enjoyment of Exercise

Our metabolism, which can be thought of as the total number of calories required to sustain our bodily functions, is comprised of three parts:

- Our Resting Metabolic Rate
- The Thermic Effect of the food we eat
- Energy expenditure through physical activity

Your resting metabolic rate is the amount of energy your body expends while in a relaxed state, and typically accounts for approximately 70% of your total daily calorie expenditure. The thermic effect of food is simply the extra calories required to digest, absorb and metabolize the food you eat, and usually accounts for about 5% of the calories you burn each day. The remaining 25% of our calorie consumption, our physical activity level, is the metabolic component we have the most control over. If we want to increase our total metabolism, it's easy to see that we need to focus on increasing our daily physical activity level. And that means we need to get up and get moving!

However, one common hurdle many overweight people face is a dislike for exercise. We choose to sit on the couch and eat our favorite foods, rather than get out and get moving. That dread of exercising can be caused by many different thoughts and emotions. For some, exercise means sweating, huffing and puffing. Others find it extremely boring. Some people even don't like to been seen exercising.

When I examined my own dislike for exercise, I realized that I had no problem with exercising with other people. I loved hiking with my friends, playing tennis, and taking yoga classes. But as soon as I thought about walking alone outside in my own neighborhood, the resistance would flare up immediately. I tapped for everything from not liking to put on lace up shoes, to not wanting to be seen by people. I had a real problem with people in cars seeing me walk by myself (hey, like the song says, nobody walks in LA!).

I finally realized that I could get at the real reason I didn't like walking alone outside by actually doing it, and tapping during the moments which caused me the most anxiety. So I did a little pre-tapping, laced up my sneakers and headed outside. I was doing fine until I got to the traffic signal at the corner. Something about making all those cars stop, and then feeling them judging me as I was about to walk across the crosswalk caused me some real discomfort. So as I stood at the crosswalk waiting for the light to change, I did some tapping on my collar bone point, without saying a word. At that moment, I was very in touch with whatever feelings were causing my resistance to walking alone, and I was able to bring my anxiety level down to a zero. As I traversed the crosswalk, I looked at people in their cars, and kind of enjoyed the power of actually making them stop in order to let me pass. It was a great moment. I was able to dissolve my resistance to walking alone. I now try to walk for at least 45 minutes 4 to 5 times a week. And my weekend hiking with friends is now just an added bonus.

Let's take a look now at any resistance you might be having to exercising. When you think about going to the gym, or taking a walk, or doing aerobics, what thoughts come up right away? Is it too hard? Do you hate sweating and being out of breath? Do you dislike that "needing a shower" feeling? Are you afraid of being seen or judged by other people while you work out? Imagine yourself beginning to exercise. What about that image feels unappealing? List your thoughts below:

When I think about exercise, the following thoughts pop into my head:

_____

_____

_____

_____

_____

Begin tapping for the insights you gained above. When you've finished, here are some other possible set up phrases to tap on:

KC   Even though I don't like exercise, I deeply and completely love and accept myself.

KC   Even though I hate to exercise, I choose to deeply and completely love and accept myself and my body.

KC   Even though I dread exercising, I choose to deeply and completely love and accept all of me.

EB   Even though I resist exercising because _____
SE   Exercise is so hard
UE   Exercise feels like work
UN   Even though exercise is sweaty
CH   And I hate getting hot and sweaty
CB   I hate huffing and puffing
UA   Even though exercise bores me to tears
TH   Even though I'd rather be watching TV instead

EB   Even though I resist going to the gym
SE   Because I don't like how I look in my gym clothes
UE   I hate working out in front of people
UN   I don't like being watched when I work out
CH   I don't like people judging me
CB   I choose to see that exercise is healthy for me
UA   I choose to embrace being healthy
TH   I now choose to commit to improving my health

EB   Even though I hate that I have to exercise, while other people are naturally slender
SE   It's not fair that I have to exercise to keep the weight off
UE   I am willing to allow my body to move more
UN   I am willing to find a way of moving that I enjoy
CH   I choose to live an active lifestyle
CB   I choose to find a fun, creative way to exercise
UA   I choose to feel vibrant and alive
TH   I choose to lovingly take care of my body from now on

Congratulations on tapping out your resistance to exercise! You should now find it much easier to get up and get moving. But if you should encounter any resistance along the way, just stop and examine your feelings and tap on them on the spot. Or simply get quiet and be with your feelings, while tapping on the 8 tapping points. You'll be enjoying physical activity again in no time. In the next chapter you'll learn the skills you'll need to be a thin person permanently!

Chapter 10

The New Thin You

Now that you're at the end of the tapping program, you may notice that you've begun to "forget" about your eating binges. You may have stopped obsessing about food and planning your meals in advance. That's great! You're beginning to have a normal relationship with food. Suddenly you're excited about your life, and are interested in doing things other than bingeing on your favorite snacks. The weight will now begin to come off, and you'll begin to feel more hopeful and more fully engaged in your own life. And now that you've discovered what a great tool EFT can be in your life, I invite you to use it all the time to address any uncomfortable memories that may pop up, for any daily annoyances that occur, or any emotional upsets you may have in your career or relationships. I still use EFT every time I realize I'm feeling discomfort of some sort. It's an amazing tool.

I mentioned earlier that food addicts use food as their primary method of stress reduction. We've seen how effective EFT can be at relieving stress and anxiety, but there are many other ways to reduce stress too. Eating and watching hours of TV are two very unproductive methods for reducing stress. They ruin your health in the long run, and prevent you from engaging fully in your life. Here are some wonderful healthy stress reduction techniques that I recommend for anyone.

Healthy Stress Reduction Techniques

Meditation is a great way to center your consciousness, and bring you fully back to yourself. Meditation is really just about quieting the mind long enough for a deep peace and relaxation to settle into your body. It can take the form of closed-eyed deep breathing, or simply visualizing a beautiful scene and immersing yourself in it. You can even meditate with a mantra, which is just any word that has deep meaning for you and is a way to keep your mind focused. It can be a word like Om, God, Jesus, Peace, or Love; whatever holds meaning for you and makes you happy is the right mantra for you. The peace, tranquility and expansiveness you feel inside when your buzzing thoughts turn off can be quite delicious.

One of my favorite types of meditation is meditation on loving kindness. This quality of loving kindness is called "metta" in the ancient far eastern Pali language. The metta meditation technique comes from the Buddhist tradition. This type of meditation not only quiets the mind and reduces stress, but it also fosters the feeling of loving acceptance of ourselves, our loved ones, the world, and even our enemies. It's very powerful.

Here is how it's done. First, sit in a comfortable position, either lotus style on the floor (cross legged, spine erect), or on a nice cushion, or in a comfortable chair. Traditionally, metta meditation begins with offering loving kindness to ourselves. Some people at the beginning of their practice may have difficulty generating that feeling toward themselves straight out of the chute.

If that's the case, you may begin by thinking of someone that you love dearly, and have no negative emotion toward. This can be a dear friend, a child, or other family member that you have great affection for, but no negative associations with. The person should be living. Many people often choose to begin with their pets, because they have an unconditional love for them. Often we can have very mixed emotions with parents, siblings or significant others, so it's best not to begin with them. Don't choose anyone for whom you feel any sexual attraction. Select someone who causes you to feel great warmth and love when you think of them. After a while, you will be easily able to begin your practice starting with yourself.

But for now, we'll begin with your loved one. Now close your eyes and take some deep cleansing breaths. Think about this person and how much you love them. Think about how much you care for this person and wish them every good thing. Feel the warmth of your love radiating outward. Allow yourself to feel this love deep within your heart. Mentally say to yourself the following phrases:

May you be safe and protected.
May you be peaceful and happy.
May you be healthy and strong.
May you have ease of well being.

Repeat these phrases mentally for a few minutes (about 3-5 to start with), until you have built up the feeling of loving kindness in your heart center. There's no need to force the feeling. Gentle intention is enough. With practice, the feeling will come more easily and naturally, and become more noticeable.

Next, direct that feeling of loving kindness toward yourself. Mentally repeat the 4 phrases:

May I be safe and protected.
May I be peaceful and happy.
May I be healthy and strong.
May I have ease of well being.

Repeat theses phrases for a few minutes, really allowing yourself to marinate in the feelings of love, peace and acceptance. When you are ready to move on, choose another loved one. This person should be someone that you have great respect for, has been good to you, and has always been there for you – like a benefactor or mentor. Repeat the 4 phrases again and send your loving kindness out to that person.

May you be safe and protected.
May you be peaceful and happy.
May you be healthy and strong.
May you have ease of well being.

After a few minutes, extend that loving kindness to someone you are completely neutral about. It could be the bank teller, a cashier at the grocery store, or even your neighbor that you wave to in passing. Repeat the four phrases for another 3 minutes or so.

After a few minutes, move on and extend your loving kindness to someone you have difficulty with, or someone you have a mild dislike for. There's no need to start with the most challenging person in your life, although with practice you will be able to do even that. Offer this person your loving kindness for a few minutes, mentally repeating the phrases above. We're offering our kindness with the understanding that every person suffers in their own way. This isn't about our approval or judgment of the person, it is about our sincere wish for the wellbeing of another. We all share the common experience of being human, and we all just want to be happy. Focus your attention and loving kindness on this person for a few minutes.

Finally, we will extend our loving kindness to the whole world - to all living beings. Continue repeating the following phrases mentally for a few minutes.

May all beings be safe and protected.
May all beings be peaceful and happy.
May all beings be healthy and strong.
May all beings have ease of well being.

When you are complete, gently open your eyes and notice the feeling of peace and balance that has taken up residence within you. With practice you'll be able to carry this feeling of peace and tranquility with you for longer and longer periods of time. The health and emotional benefits of this practice are many, including increased peace, serenity, clarity of thought, as well as a radiant inner beauty that no amount of makeup can reproduce! Try it. I promise it will change your life.

Relaxing Activities

If you prefer a relaxing activity to meditation, you can always call a positive and supportive friend. Don't call a negative Nelly, because they will only cause you more stress. If you don't have any positive friends, find some. Positive friendships have been shown to increase our health, longevity and overall happiness. I have a friend that I can telephone or skype with for 3 or 4 hours, and it's like no time has passed at all. If you don't have someone available to talk to, then talk to yourself. Write your thoughts down on paper. Some people find journaling to be very relaxing.

Not to mention, it can be a great tool for getting in touch with any feelings that could really use some tapping.

One of the best ways to relax is through some kind of physical activity. The exertion of exercise releases endorphins, the body's own natural antidepressants. Endorphins are chemicals that are produced in the brain when we exercise, or are in love, and have an effect similar to opioid drugs. They give us a sense of increased energy and wellbeing. No doubt you've heard of "runner's high" before. Long distance runners frequently extol the pleasures of the high that they receive from their runs.

I personally find exercise just for the sake of exercise to be less fun than if I combine it with things that I already enjoy. I'm very social and I enjoy talking with my friends. So it's very easy for me to walk a couple of miles without noticing it while talking with my friends about my favorite subjects. And if I combine that with the beauty of nature, well then I've got a home run. Some people may call it hiking, but I call it having a conversation while enjoying nature. I also love to dance, so shaking my booty to the radio while I clean house is natural, organic fun. I also love to stretch my body by doing yoga while listening to a native American flute CD. It makes me feel very invigorated, yet relaxed, calm and centered. I think yoga is perhaps the perfect exercise. It's not too sweaty, and it can keep you strong, flexible and healthy well into old age!

You as a Thin Person

Now that you have cleared out the barriers to your weight loss, you're well on your way to becoming the slender person you want to be. You're about to enter the ranks of the thin and healthy. As it turns out, thin people think differently than overweight people. As a formerly overweight person, you probably remember what it was like to be obsessed with food. You were always pre-occupied with when your next meal was coming, and what you were going to eat. You might have even planned your meals farther in advance than just later in the day. I know I did. But thin people don't think like that.

Thin people are generally unconcerned about their next meal, since they're too busy living their lives. They also tend not to judge whether a particular food is good or bad or has too many calories, they just eat it without getting hung up on the guilt. People with food issues tend to agonize over whether a particular food is good or bad. Thin people don't. They eat what they want. They just eat it in moderate quantities. Plus, they stop eating before they get to the point of being too full. Food addicts are so far out of touch with their bodies and emotions, that the only signal for them to stop eating is the physical discomfort of being overly full.

Releasing your food addiction may feel like completely new territory for you. While it's very exciting, and all things are now possible for you, you may not currently have a reference point for how to actually be a thin person. Thin people not only think differently about food, but they also have different values, behaviors and habits than food addicts. We're going to explore some of the ways thin people see the world differently and how you can develop their healthy habits which will serve you the rest of your life.

Ever since Dr Maxwell Maltz published his bestseller "Psycho-Cybernetics" in 1960, it has been generally accepted in the mental health field that it takes about 21 days for us to establish a new

245

habit. After which time, it actually becomes harder to go against the newly formed habit than to continue doing it. So if you can stick with following your new healthy habits each day for at least 3 weeks, you are well on your way to having them for life.

We already addressed resistance to exercise earlier. Even though you will no longer be depriving yourself of, or bingeing on particular foods, at the end of the day, your body mass is still essentially a mathematical equation. You need to take in equal or fewer calories to the number of calories you burn in order not to gain weight. Keeping the weight off becomes harder as we get older, and our metabolism naturally slows down a little. Also, the vast majority of our jobs today involve some kind of desk work. Earlier in my career, I worked at a lot of administrative jobs which kept me sitting in a chair in my cubicle for hours on end. I felt like a veal calf being prepared for slaughter, not being able to move about freely. During that time, I packed on the pounds pretty rapidly.

Because our modern society has created so many time and labor saving devices, we don't move around as much as our ancestors did. All that sitting for hours at a time allows our muscles to atrophy. And our muscle cells are our body's chief calorie burners. A muscle cell burns roughly 3 times the calories that the average fat cell burns. Muscles are our body's calorie burning powerhouses. So, the less muscle mass we have, the fatter we get. It's simple math. The good news is the more we move, the more muscle we build, and the more fat we burn. Consequently, regular physical activity will become your secret weapon for keeping excess weight off.

You'd be amazed at how few calories a body at rest really requires. Consider that skeletal muscles burn about 13 calories per kilogram (1kg = about 2.2 lbs) per day. Also consider that on the average, 36% of a woman's body mass is muscle, and 42% for men. If we do a little math, we see that for a 180 lb adult, our muscles burn about 379 calories for women and 442 calories just sitting around each day. Of course this doesn't take into account the paltry calories per day that your fat cells will burn. But it does illustrate how a desk job combined with a diet of fast food combo meals, averaging well over 1,000 calories a piece, can be a recipe for obesity.

The Chinese have a great saying, "If the legs are healthy, then the body is healthy." That is why in some parts of the world you can see large groups of adults in parks each day practicing tai chi, or taking long walks, to keep their legs and bodies in tip top shape. Walking in itself is a weight bearing exercise. You're walking around holding 120 to 200 lbs aloft! In the practice of chilel chi gong there is an exercise called a "wall squat" aimed directly at keeping the muscles in the legs and glutes in optimum working order.

If you've ever noticed, older people don't really begin declining in health until they stop moving. The newspapers are full of stories about octogenarians who still dance, or garden, or do yoga every day. It's the aches and pains brought on by poor diet and sedentary living that eventually catch up to people, causing them to become less and less mobile. Convalescent homes are designed for the express purpose of getting the aged out of bed and moving again. So for your own health and longevity – keep moving!

Positive Engagement

Another trait thin people share is that they have hobbies and activities to engage in other than just eating. They keep themselves quite busy, until all of a sudden hunger will sneak up on them. They almost resent the time they have to take away from their activities to sit down and eat. Take a second and think about how engaged you are in your own life. How much TV do you watch during the average week? How much time do you spend online? For most people, watching television is an escape from the reality that their lives are a disappointment. It's a way to feel like you're having an exciting life - by watching others have an exciting life. But really, if you're watching several hours a night, you're probably not really having a life at all. And if you're single, these solitary indoor activities also tend to keep you isolated from your community. They keep you from meeting new and interesting people and potential new friends.

The first time I ever understood what the term "in the flow" meant, was when I was learning how to do enameling (glass art on metal, involving a kiln). A friend of a friend was instructing me, and I decided to make a pendant for my sister for her birthday. I started at about 10 in the morning, and by 5 o'clock that evening I found I couldn't - didn't want to - stop. I finally had to, because I had previous dinner plans with friends. But the point was that I had found something SO absorbing, so creatively fulfilling, that I could have done it for hours non-stop.

If you really want to LIVE, think about the things in your life that you return to over and over again in your thoughts and conversations with friends. Those are your passions. Also, think about the following questions. What did you love doing as a child? Did you like to ride horses? Did you love to read science fiction? Were you an avid knitter or crocheter? How do you express your creativity now on a daily basis? Creative expression is a well known contributor to one's overall happiness. Being creative, intellectually curious, and contributing to the world at large give our lives meaning and purpose.

Think about revisiting some of the hobbies you had as a youngster. Or consider volunteering in some capacity using your unique skills to help improve other people's lives. There are also organizations all over the place that have free lectures and meetings. And with the internet at your disposal, it's easier than ever to find a group of people interested in the same things that make your own heart sing. One of my dear friends joined an amateur astronomy club, and now has access to borrowing from a network of impressive telescopes - for free. She couldn't be happier! So what I'm saying is, make the commitment to yourself to make this year the one where you start doing things that you really love. Make this the year you really start living!

Re-Learning How to Eat: Now What?

Thin people also eat differently than food addicts. First, they eat more slowly. Addicts have a tendency to chew quickly and gulp their food, almost in a daze. Frequently they eat in front of the TV, in the car, or anywhere besides the kitchen table. Food addicts eat in kind of a zombie-like trance, and keep stuffing the food in their mouths until all of it is gone, or until their stomach hurts. Whichever comes first.

Part of becoming a thin person involves eating more consciously. It means paying attention to what and how we're eating. We should try and be fully present when we eat, without multitasking and distractions, like watching television or reading a book. We should ideally sit at our dining table, bring our consciousness to the present moment and focus on the smell, flavor and texture of the food we are enjoying. Whatever food you happen to be eating, enjoy it fully without any guilt or recrimination. Eating in this way will help you release your old habits of inhaling your food unconsciously and going back for more without a second thought. Anything we enjoy is worth doing slowly and consciously, giving it our full attention - and eating a meal is no different. The quality and quantity of the food we eat is a direct reflection of the respect we have for ourselves and our body.

I used to have a boyfriend who took forever to finish his meals. He was also as thin as a rail. I could swear he was counting how many times he chewed, but I couldn't prove it. But there is a certain amount of wisdom in how he ate. Eating slowly and deliberately accomplishes a couple of things. First it allows us to completely break up the food and maximize its surface area, allowing for better digestion and nutrient utilization. There are enzymes in our saliva that aid in digestion. For example, ptyalin is an enzyme which helps break down starchy foods into a simple sugar that our body can then metabolize for energy. The more we chew our food, the more these helpful enzymes come into contact with the molecules in our food. Eating slowly also gives the body time to signal that it is satisfied.

Growing up, your mother may have told you to chew your food 30 times before you swallow. As an experiment, count how many times you currently chew a bite of food before swallowing. When you get an average, now try lengthening the amount of time you chew eat bite. Try increasing the number of times you chew before swallowing. The ideal number of times to chew is not a hard and fast rule, due to the differing density and textures of various types of food. But a handy guideline is to chew until you can no longer identify the type of food in your mouth by its texture. We're going for a pasty consistency here. If you can still tell you are chewing a piece of steak, or you can identify that stalk of celery by its crunch, you haven't chewed enough. Chewing that long may feel a little weird at first, but after a while, it will become your new normal. Chewing thoroughly will maximize the nutritional benefits of everything you eat, and take unnecessary stress off your digestive system.

Also, there's evidence which indicates that eating slowly may also lengthen your life. The longest lived people in the world seem to be concentrated in the area of the islands of Okinawa Japan. The researchers behind the Okinawa Centenarian Study (people over the age of one hundred) found, as you might expect, that this population appeared very healthy, remained very active, and ate a vegetable and fruit rich diet. In addition, they also shared the common cultural practice of hara hachi bu, which roughly translated means, "eat only until you are 80 percent full". This practice amounts to de facto calorie restriction, which is a theory currently receiving much interest from the scientific community for its effect of increasing longevity in lab animals.

It's hypothesized that reduced caloric intake results in reduced generation of the free radicals which are responsible for cellular ageing. Even if we don't choose to practice caloric restriction, we can take a page out of the playbook of these thriving centenarians by beginning the habit of only eating until we are 80% full, and then waiting 20 minutes to see if we are still hungry before going back for seconds.

Another intriguing concept to come out of the field of nutrition is something called volumetrics. Barbara Rolls, Ph.D., a nutrition and obesity researcher at Penn State University observed through her work that it's the volume of food we eat, rather than the number of calories we consume that causes us to experience satiety or fullness. She also noticed that people have a tendency to eat the same quantity of food each day regardless of how many calories they consume. From her findings she extrapolated that we can eat the same quantity of food by substituting foods with fewer calories (lower calorie density) for ones with higher calories (high calorie density) without experiencing hunger.

On her volumetrics eating plan, Dr. Rolls suggests eating the weight of food that you normally would, but swap out high calorie foods containing sugar and fat for those that contain a lot of water and fiber, both of which increase our sense of fullness. Some of the beneficial foods she suggests are ones you might expect to find in a healthy eating plan such as; fruit, vegetables, whole grains, legumes, low-fat dairy, fish and skinless poultry. Likewise, things to be avoided would be; full fat dairy, sodas, starches and sweets. Her plan does allow the occasional treat, as does any reasonable eating plan, but Dr. Rolls admonishes that it is important to stay under your daily caloric recommendations. Her way of eating is not really new, but the idea that we can retain the volume of our food intake, while reducing our caloric intake and not experience hunger is noteworthy. You certainly can't do any harm by eating healthier foods in any event! So to sum up, eating thin involves:

1. Eating consciously, without distractions. Enjoy your food.
2. Chewing thoroughly to increase digestive effectiveness.
3. Stopping at 80% fullness to see if you're still hungry.
4. If you are still hungry 20 minutes later, have more.

5.   Maximize your intake of whole foods, and minimize processed foods.

The point of eating this way is never deprivation. The point is to honor your body with both the amount and nutritional quality of the foods you eat. Knowing that you always have the freedom to go back for more if your body requires it, will keep you from feeling deprived.

Listening to Your Body

As you release your food addiction and stop obsessing over food, you'll be freed up to take your eating cues from how your body truly feels. The "three square meals a day" food model, with its large plates of food and in between meal snacks, is simply a construct of modern society. It forces us to prepare and consume large meals at pre-determined times each day – whether we are actually hungry or not. Our pre-historic ancestors did not eat this way, nor do animals in the wild.

In fact, some nutritionists claim that it's much better to eat 6 small meals a day instead of 3 large ones. As I mentioned earlier, recent scientific studies have shown that caloric restriction in lab animals has the effect of increasing their longevity. The new data has even spawned a whole "caloric restriction for longevity" movement. Now, I'm not saying we should starve ourselves. I'm simply saying that we need far less food to thrive than we've been taught by television advertising and the "super sized" fast food chain restaurants. I think that's fairly evident given the obesity epidemic both in the United States and western world in general.

I'm also suggesting that we learn to listen to our body's wisdom and only eat when we are hungry and not by the numbers on the clock. If we listen, our body will also tell us what it wants to eat in order to give it the nutrients it requires. For example, I sometimes find myself craving sushi rolls for iodine, or a baked yam for beta carotene. I'm always amazed at the wisdom of my body, and I try to pay attention to what it has to tell me.

As an experiment, you can designate one day where you have no predetermined agenda to eat whatsoever. On that day, commit to only eating when your stomach signals you it's time. When you feel yourself getting hungry, ask your body what it needs for its optimum health at that moment, and eat that. This exercise will help you get in tune with your body's hunger signals. You may find that your body doesn't want 3 full meals with snacks in between. You may want 2 small meals in the morning and at dinner, with a larger lunch. You may prefer to have a small glass of fresh juice first thing in the morning with a big salad for lunch and a smaller dinner. Whatever your body wants is right for you. The point is not to restrict your eating, but to be relaxed about it. Become conscious of when, how much, and what your body wants to eat, and honor that.

Better Food = Better Health

My diet now consists primarily of organic fruits, vegetables, nuts and seeds. I try and limit my intake of meat, dairy, wheat and grains (many grains contain gluten, which generates an inflammatory response within the body). As a result, I am experiencing better health than I have at any other time in my life. I also try to eat my produce raw whenever possible, and occasionally bake or steam my vegetables. But even though I strive to eat as healthy and nutritiously as I can, I still allow myself a sweet indulgence whenever I want one.

However, I found over time that the cleaner I ate, the less I actually craved any sort of junk food. The more high carbohydrate foods I consumed, the more I found myself craving them. Now I actually look forward to the flavors of ripe, juicy fruits and organic, brightly colored vegetables. I just love the feeling of all those vital nutrients coursing through my veins. Junk food just doesn't taste all that good to me anymore. So when I do choose to indulge, I tend to reach for purer, higher quality foods, like a piece of rich, organic dark chocolate. In which case, just a little bit of such an indulgent treat satisfies my taste buds. I no longer need to eat a pound bar of chocolate to satisfy an emotional craving.

I would also encourage everyone consider reducing their meat intake, while increasing their intake of organic plant-based foods. If you feel inspired to do so, try and eat more of your vegetables in their raw state to retain more of their natural vitamins, amino acids and enzymes. If you're afraid of not getting enough "protein", you simply have to look at our closest animal relatives, the great apes. Gorillas and chimpanzees maintain their sizeable mass eating only plants. The same is true for elephants and giraffes. These big creatures are living proof that large mammals do not require "meat" protein in order to thrive.

What is protein anyway? A protein is really just a chain of amino acids that the body must first break down in order to make use of them for cellular metabolism. According to the US Institute of Medicine, out of the total 20 amino acids, there are 9 which cannot be synthesized in the human body and must be obtained through our food. Meat and dairy are usually considered "complete" proteins in that they contain all 9 of the essential amino acids.

Plant foods, as a whole, generally contain varying percentages of the necessary amino acids. But some, like soy, quinoa, amaranth, buckwheat, nutritional yeast, and spirulina are considered complete proteins in their own right. However, by eating a variety of different types of fruits, vegetables, beans, legumes and nuts, it's easy to get an adequate supply of all the essential amino acids without consuming animal products.

Many Americans may be familiar with the original food pyramid designed by the United States Department of Agriculture in 1992. This approach to eating emphasized far too much bread, cereal, pasta, meat and dairy, and has since been revised. The pyramid was updated in 2005 to include a larger percentage of fresh fruits and vegetables. Research studies have shown a link between the consumption of animal products and disease. One of the largest and most comprehensive studies, the Cornell-Oxford China study, showed a clear correlation between consumption of meat and dairy products and chronic degenerative diseases such as cancer, coronary artery disease, osteoporosis and diabetes.

In fact, ingesting too much protein can even have negative consequences. Excess amino acids which are consumed but are unneeded by the body must be processed through the kidneys and expelled in your urine, causing an increased burden on the kidneys. Plus, many of us believe we need more protein than we actually do. The amount of protein our bodies require varies, and is heavily dependent upon our daily activity level. The World Health Organization recommends a daily intake of approximately .8 grams of protein for every kilogram of body weight, or roughly .36 grams per pound. So if your ideal weight is 125 lbs, then you would need to eat approximately 45 grams of protein per day. That's a fairly easy amount to achieve. Of course if you're more active, like a weight lifter or marathon runner, you would require more per pound. To show you how easy it is to achieve the recommended level of protein consumption, consider the protein contents of the following foods:

Protein Source	gms
3 oz chicken breast	29
1 cup lowfat 1 % cottage cheese	28
1 scoop (28 gm) soy protein isolate	25
3 oz top sirloin	23
3 oz broiled salmon	23
1 cup boiled soybeans	22
1 ground beef patty	21
3 oz canned tuna (water packed)	21
1 cup lentils	18
1 cup beans (pinto, black, kidney)	12
1 cup chickpeas	12
8 oz plain lowfat yogurt	12
1 cup soymilk	10
1/2 cup tofu	10
2 T hemp seeds	10
1 cup lowfat 2% milk	8
2 T peanut butter	8
1 hard boiled egg	6
1 oz almonds	6
1 cup cooked brown rice	5
2 T tahini (sesame seed butter)	5
1 oz walnuts	4
1 cup broccoli	3

When choosing your protein, you should consider the quality of the source. Most livestock today are pumped full of hormones and antibiotics which are then passed along to us when we eat them. So if you are a meat eater, you should always try and choose organic or kosher meats when possible. Or even better, try getting more of your daily protein intake from plant sources. As you can see from the chart on the previous page, many of the beans and soy products rival meat in protein content.

I also happen to believe there is an energetic component to food as well. A fruit picked fresh off the tree will be filled with more life force and nutrients than the typical store bought apple which can be months old. And if you really think about it, meat is a food that is already in the decomposition process by the time we receive it. We all know what happens to a cadaver, and how rapidly it will start to decompose if left alone in the open air. Meat begins to rot as soon as the animal is slaughtered. Meat truly is a "dead" food. So I invite you think about getting more of your protein from healthy plant sources like beans and legumes, and raw, sprouted seeds.

I guarantee if you adopt the diet and lifestyle changes mentioned in this chapter, you'll experience an abundant increase in your overall health. I made these changes myself and they've made all the difference in my life. I'm experiencing my best health in over 20 years. I challenge you to commit to caring for yourself and honoring your body every day. Feed your body healthy, nourishing foods, and get enough exercise, play and rest each and every day. You deserve it!

Chapter 11

Beyond Your Wildest Dreams

Now that you've tapped on many of your limiting thoughts and emotions, you're probably beginning to feel a sense of peace and freedom that you've never felt before. You've taken powerful steps to release yourself from the grip of compulsive eating and food addiction by eliminating your emotional blocks to permanent weight loss. But what may not be as readily apparent is that at the same time, you've also rooted out the negative emotions and beliefs that were blocking you from living a life of happiness, renewed passion and total abundance. This new feeling of possibility will allow you to begin to pursue your dreams with a new vitality. Part two of the Thinstead process focuses on how you can create a life of joy and excitement.

Increasing Your Happiness Quotient

All human beings strive to be happy. In fact, we spend our whole lives trying to obtain pleasure and avoid pain. But "pleasure" is really just a mood state we derive from external things and circumstances. And since pleasure is entirely dependent upon us having the things or circumstances we want, pleasure seeking as a strategy leaves us vulnerable to unhappiness as soon as things don't go our way. When we live our lives externally like that, we set ourselves up for unhappiness. That's because life has a tendency to throw us curveballs. And when we can only be happy when our circumstances are pleasant, or because we bought that new purse we've been eyeing, that also means whenever we get a speeding ticket or lose that promotion we're no longer happy.

What most people don't realize is that happiness is fundamentally an internal process. So in order for us to be enduringly happy, we have to pay attention to what's going on inside us.

Happiness Is An Inside Job

One of my greatest inspirations and role models is a man called Lester Levenson, who is considered by many to be a modern spiritual master. In the early 1950's, Lester suffered his second heart attack. Cardiology back then wasn't as advanced as it is today, and Lester was sent home with some medication and was told he should not expect to improve. He was admonished not to strain himself in any way, and try to lead a life of inactivity. Deeply depressed, Lester contemplated suicide by pills using his medications. However, reasoning that he could kill himself later if he wanted, he decided to start inquiring into the meaning of his life, and how he had gotten to where he now found himself.

At first he read all the books on philosophy he could get his hands on, but found no answers contained in them. He finally realized that all the answers to his questions were only to be found inside himself. One of the questions he asked was "What is happiness?" Lester pondered this question and began making a mental inventory of all the times he had been happiest in his life. At first he thought it might have been when he had been loved. He thought about the various women in his life and the love he had shared with each of them.

But then he thought back on being in the hospital and how he could see that he was very much loved by his family and friends. In fact, even before he was hospitalized, Lester had been loved, and yet he had still not been happy. It was now obvious to Lester that being loved was not the answer, but it was rather the love that he **GAVE** that had made him happy. It was the love he gave to others which had made him truly joyful. Lester had discovered the true way to lasting happiness – giving love. Not only did Lester end up living for another 42 years despite his heart condition diagnosis, he also dedicated the rest of his life to sharing his knowledge with the world. His legacy lives on today in the teachings contained in the Sedona Method and many others.

Do you ever wonder why we feel so good around babies and our pets? Do you know why spending time with them lowers our blood pressure and gives us a sense of wellbeing? It's because we love them unconditionally. It's because we want nothing from them. We only want to shower them with our love and affection, without expecting anything whatsoever in return. Babies and pets are little mirrors that show us the boundless love waiting inside us. That kind of unconditional love is the closest thing we humans have to heaven on earth.

I myself had a cat named Binks for over 15 years whom I absolutely loved. Binks used to follow me all over the house, and even sat on my lap while I watched TV in the evenings. When she died, I was absolutely devastated. For a few years after that, whenever I allowed myself to think of her, I would weep. Then one day I finally realized that Binks wasn't really the one doing anything in our relationship, but in fact, it was **my love for her**, that I missed. I wasn't really grieving for her company so much as I was grieving for my lost opportunity to love completely and unreservedly each and every day.

Sometimes we find it easier to love our pets and babies because we don't expect anything from them. They haven't hurt us in the ways other people in our lives have. It seems tougher to love people because there are egos involved – both ours and theirs. It may seem difficult at first, but it's vital that we learn to love everyone, without judgment, if we are to achieve true inner peace. We should learn to forgive and love others not for their benefit - but because it is good for US.

Cultivating Love in Your Life

There are a number of ways in which we can cultivate more love in our life. Two superb ways are through prayer and meditation. Prayer brings us closer to our Creator, our Divine Source. The practice of meditation stills our mind, and silences our thoughts long enough to get in touch with our true essence - Divine Love. Both practices center us and return us to ourselves. I highly encourage everyone to find time each day to spend time in prayer or meditation. Your happiness level, as well as your health, will be greatly increased for it.

As I mentioned earlier, you can also choose to spend more time with animals and babies. They both allow us to tap into the love that is already dwelling inside us. You can also try incorporating more nature into your life. Whether that means going for a morning or evening walk, hiking with friends, spending time at the beach, camping or just gardening, being in touch with Mother Earth is very restorative to our soul.

Another great way to cultivate love is to use your time, talents and abilities to help others. You can volunteer your time or services for free for the benefit of others. You can volunteer for a charity or other cause you believe in. What skills do you have that you can put to use in service to others? Do you love to cook? You could volunteer to cook at your nearest homeless shelter. Are you a good writer? Offer to help a non-profit organization create marketing materials. Are you a lawyer or mechanic? Offer your services for free to a few people each month who really could use the help. The point here is to offer your skills to help others and the world.

Doing Your Work With Love

But even when we aren't busy volunteering, we can still choose to bring love into the present moment of whatever we're doing. The way we do that is to perform all of our tasks with the spirit of love. You probably already experience this when you're making dinner for your family. The love and caring you feel for your family makes its way into the food you serve them. You're preparing the meal with love. You can bring that same love to all your daily activities if you choose. For example, when you brush your teeth, think of how you are caring for your teeth, and how you love and appreciate them for all the hard work they do for you each day. When you're at work, dealing with your coworkers and customers, send the intention that your work blesses them and prospers them in their lives. Doing your work with love creates more satisfaction in your life.

Our work becomes even more satisfying when we enjoy it and when it makes use of our greatest talents. I once read an article that talked about the distinction between work and toil. Work is performing an activity which produces a result. It's kind of neutral. Then there's toil. Toil is working at something you actively dislike. Do you love what you do? Maybe not. Are there some aspects of it that you do each day that you do enjoy, or make you feel confident, satisfied and fulfilled? I discovered that I really liked the helping aspect of most of my jobs. I loved fulfilling my customers and coworkers needs. That part of my job gave me immense satisfaction.

Think about the parts of your job that you enjoy doing. Is there any way you could do MORE of that? Is there any way you could do less of what you don't like? Could you trade with a coworker for something she dislikes, but you would enjoy? Maybe your work is just not really your cup of tea, and you've been toying with the idea of changing your career. I know how you feel. I struggled with the question "What do I want to do with my life?" for many years. And I think that the reason so many of us can't identify what we want to do with our lives is that we've had so little practice in getting what we want from life that we don't even bother having preferences or desires any more. I know that was definitely part of my problem.

Manifesting Your Destiny

Most personally fulfilled people today accept that we shape our own reality. The wildly successful book and DVD "The Secret" is evidence that people everywhere resonate to the essential truth contained in the Law of Attraction. It's easy to see how, in our own lives, we attract more of whatever we focus our attention on. I was introduced to the law of attraction in the 1990's when a dear friend gave me a set of Abraham Hicks cassettes. At the time, it was new information for me, but it changed the way I looked at my life forever.

I was immediately drawn to the idea of being able to shape my own destiny. But for years I struggled with the material, trying to figure out how to make my dreams come true. And I think that many people who are newly introduced to the concept of the law of attraction feel the same way. I was struggling with what my life purpose was, and what my career should be. I had mainly held well paid administrative jobs, and I was very good at them, but I still felt like something was missing.

Like Thoreau, Dr. Wayne Dyer warns us not to "die with our music still inside us". I was determined to live a life of purpose and fulfillment, but was frustrated by not knowing what my purpose was. After much reflection, I finally realized that our life's purpose and passion may not emerge as a clear career path or declared college major. Sometimes it makes itself known as an interest or hobby that follows us throughout our lives. Sometimes it can even be a topic of conversation that we return to over and over again with our friends. Or it can also be the culmination of the journey we've taken in our lives, like when Candy Lightner, a grieving mother, founded Mothers Against Drunk Driving in her deceased daughter's honor.

For me, I had a lifelong fascination with metaphysics and holistic health. I could easily remember what herbs and vitamins were good for what ailments, and I was constantly giving friends and family nutritional advice. I also enrolled in oriental medicine and acupuncture school, became a certified Reiki practitioner, a hypnotherapist, and investigated many other healing systems. But I was still confused about how I could best use my talents and interests to help others. I kept dancing around the idea of holistic health, but it seemed I couldn't find my direction. Then one day I discovered EFT, and it was the most powerful healing modality I had ever seen. From that point on, I knew I wanted to help people overcome their anxiety, depression, addictions and physical ailments in order to live a better life.

In my practice, I see many people like I was - people who don't know what they want from life. They don't have any passions, or any idea about what career path they want to pursue. More often than not, this stunting of passion and desire stems from not being able to have what they wanted as children. It comes from having had their dreams unknowingly crushed by loved ones and authority figures. But once they use EFT to release their sadness over having their desires stifled, they usually spring back to life and start really living and fulfilling their precious dreams. It happened that way for me, when the idea for ThinStead came to me like a flash of lightning. It was so obvious really. ThinStead was the natural expression of my desire to help others live their best lives, combined with my own weight loss journey, plus the most effective healing modality I had ever encountered. And so I ask you to take a look at your own interests, your favorite topics, and your life's journey and see if you might be able to combine them into the career of your dreams.

You CAN Have it All

Besides coming to understand that having my dreams truly was possible, another thing that made the law of attraction really click for me was the realization that no struggle was actually necessary. What that means is, we don't have to plan, or scheme, or figure out HOW to "get" our desires. That's not our job. Our only job is to set forth our desires and wait for the Universe to answer. If we are clear about our desires, and open to the possibility of receiving them, what will happen is that synchronicities will begin to show up, whether it's a sale on the exact item we want, or someone is giving away just what we are looking for, or we meet someone who has the knowledge, skill or opportunity we need. At that point we will take **inspired action**, which won't feel like a struggle to us at all. Our path will be made clear and our efforts made easy. Whenever we contemplate an action, and it feels easy and natural, we know we are living our truth. If we feel resistance in any way, it's not right for us at that moment. Lester Levenson often said that when we are in a place of happiness and love, manifestation is effortless, because we are in harmony with the tune of the Universe itself. So now the real question is...

What Do You Want?

People have a tendency to see the negative in life. They can easily tell you what it is they don't like. They hate their job, their boss, their marriage, whatever. But people seldom take time to think about what it is they DO want. If someone were to ask you what's wrong, you probably have a long list of gripes that you've been ruminating over for years. But if a genie were to pop out of a bottle and ask you what you wanted, would you be able to answer? Some people have become so used to not getting what they want in life, that they've stopped trying to have any desires at all.

If that sounds a little familiar, and you're unsure of what you really want from life, here are some tapping set ups designed to clear out the blockages to living a life full of purpose and passion:

Even though I don't know what I want from my life, I deeply and completely love and accept myself anyway.

Even though I'm not in touch with my wants and desires

Even though I haven't been able to get what I want in life

Even though I haven't ever been allowed to have what I want

Even though they never let me have what I want

Even though I haven't let myself have what I truly want

Even though because of that, I don't even know what I want from my life

Even though I learned not to have any passion or zest for life

Even though I stopped having any dreams at all, I now choose to live a life of happiness, fulfillment and passion from now on.

EB	I choose to let go of these feelings of frustration
SE	I am willing to believe my dreams can come true
UE	I choose to believe they are on their way to me now
UN	I choose to be clear about my wants and desires
CH	I choose to anticipate fun and excitement
CB	I choose to believe I deserve to be happy
UA	I love knowing that the Universe supports me
TH	I love knowing my desires are on their way to me now

Now here are some questions to help you unlock your true desires:

What if anything do you do currently to express yourself creatively? Cooking? Painting? Writing? Handicrafts? What would you do if you had more time and money?

_____

_____

_____

_____

_____

What did you used to like to do as a child? Draw? Fly kites or model airplanes? Engage in sports? Play with animals? Build forts in the woods? List them here:

_____

_____

_____

_____

_____

_____

What conversational topics do you find yourself returning to over and over again? Do you love to talk about politics, or metaphysics or the paranormal?

_____

_____

_____

_____

_____

What is it that you most want out of life? How will you know when you get it?

_____

_____

_____

_____

_____

_____

What do you think it is that stops you from getting the things you want?

_____

_____

_____

_____

_____

_____

Try and think of some solutions to your problem contained in the answer above, no matter how ludicrous. If you said money was a barrier, could your problem be solved by a sweepstakes win, an inheritance, an angel investor, an educational grant, finding a rare coin, a new job offer, or making friends with just the sort of person whose talents, knowledge and expertise you really need?

There are probably dozens of ways that your problem could be solved. The point of this exercise is learning not to put a limit on the power of the Universe to provide an infinite number of solutions to your problems. Try listing some of the many ways in which your problems could disappear, no matter how outrageous they might seem.

_____

_____

_____

_____

_____

_____

One of the most valuable ideas I came away with from the teachings of "A Course in Miracles" is the idea of "being open to the miracle". By miracle, the author is referring to the change in perception which results in the solution to our problems. I find that whenever I declare to the Universe that I'm open to the miracle, the Universe snaps into action and things start to happen very rapidly. One time when I threw my hands up in the air and shouted "I'm willing to accept the miracle!" I received a job offer the very next day. So never ever put any limitations on how the Divine Source can help you with your problems. Your Creator loves you and knows how to best give you that which you most desire. If only you will allow it.

Sometimes it feels like everyone I talk to these days hates their job. Hating your job, your boss and your coworkers seems almost like an epidemic these days. That probably accounts for why, according to Nielsen's "State of the Media" (4th Qtr 2010), Americans spend close to 5 hours a day on average watching television. And that number is on the rise. People are watching that much television in order to escape their lives, to turn their brains off and not have to think about how miserable they are. If you add up 9 to 11 hours of working at, getting ready for, and driving to a job you hate, plus 8 hours of sleep, plus another 4-5 hours of watching television, how much are you really living? It's kind of disturbing if you really sit down and think about it. Do you really want to spend your life waiting for something to happen to improve your life, or do you want to live a more meaningful and engaged life **right now**?

A famous Buddhist aphorism says that "all life is suffering". The prescription for happiness offered by the Buddhist sages is to not resist what IS. That's because there really is no future, or past for that matter, there is only the ever present now. Next week or next year don't exist. We live in the now. Even when we get to next week, we will still be living **now**. It's very dangerous to put off living your life until some magical time in the future. You end up putting both your happiness and your life off until some later date - until you lose 20 pounds, until you win the lotto, until you pay off your debts, until you get married. We can only live one moment at a time anyway - so isn't it much better to begin living a better life now, in this very moment?

Freedom to Choose

Another thing that helps you accept your current life situation, whatever it is, is to realize that you are always free to choose. I disliked one of my early office jobs for many years, until I suddenly realized that I was there by **choice**. As much as I desperately wanted out, the truth of the matter is I wanted the salary and the security it offered me MORE. I could have at any moment quit my job. But most likely my finances would have suffered as a result, or I would have had to take on a roommate. But none of the consequences of quitting my job seemed preferable to continuing to work at that drudge of a job. So I CHOSE to keep it.

273

Even if you feel trapped by your current circumstances, it's important to realize that you are choosing to do so. Remember that you are always free to quit your job, or stop paying your credit card bills, or leave that crummy relationship. You are simply not choosing that choice right now. Your life as it is now is a direct reflection of the choices you've made to date and the values that you hold. Within that realization lies a lot of power. When you accept you are always at choice, you know that you are also free to choose to live a different life and can begin drafting a plan to make it happen.

I remember reading a story about a woman who received her college degree at age 90. I was very impressed by her choice to go back to school, as well as a little envious of her courage and determinedness. Have you ever thought of changing your career in mid life, but thought "it's too late"? If so, just think about how long the next 40 to 50 years will be doing something you dislike. There are plenty of happy and fulfilled people who changed careers mid-stream. People switch careers all the time. It's the norm now for people to have multiple careers during their lifetime.

Think about it, the person we are in our teens or twenties is not the same person we are at age 45. How could we possibly have known at that age what we wanted to do for the rest of our lives? So if your heart is calling you in another direction, follow it. Because at the end of our lives, the things we regret most are not the things we did, but the things we didn't do. So be courageous and re-choose who you want to be. Re-choose a life of purpose and fulfillment.

Here are some set ups that you might find useful if you're experiencing unhappiness in your job:

Even though I dislike my job and my boss, I choose to do my best and love and accept myself completely.

Even though I'm afraid I might be stuck at this job forever and I'm really frustrated, I deeply and completely love and accept myself anyway.

Even though I don't want to try and learn to enjoy my current job, I choose to try and accept myself and my situation as it is now.

EB	I hate my job
SE	I resent the fact that I have to work there
UE	I don't want to work there anymore
UN	I don't want to work hard
CH	I want to be somewhere else right now
CB	It's not fair that I have to work there
UA	It's not fair that I have to go to a job I hate
TH	I just want to escape

EB	But I choose to learn how to be happy in the now
SE	I choose to release my resistance to my life as it is now
UE	I choose to be peaceful instead of resisting my life as it is
UN	I choose to allow myself to enjoy parts of my work day
CH	I choose to find things to be happy about during the day
CB	I choose to feel grateful for the other abundance I do have in my life already
UA	I choose see that I am always free to choose
TH	I choose to look forward to manifesting even BETTER things in my life, including a new career that deeply fulfills me

Clarity: The Key To Getting What You Really Want

Our thoughts and emotions are like a lens that focuses the power of the Universe into one small area of creation. The full manifesting power of the Universe is available to us at all times and is simply waiting for our command. So if we are feeling lack, the Universe says, "By all means, feel free to experience lack." The Universe doesn't judge what you should or shouldn't have, it just responds to your thoughts and emotions in kind. Now if you were to change your mind, and choose to experience total abundance, the Universe would respond by saying "Total abundance, coming right up!"

But as a part of this experience of physical reality, we also have the buffer of time. Which is a good thing - because if you momentarily thought of a black widow spider, you wouldn't necessarily want one to appear in your hand. So the Universe kindly allows us a little time to get our thoughts together and choose again what it is we really want. With that said, all of your thoughts are creative, and so each one attracts a particular experience into your life. So if you have had many years of lack mentality, you may still be experiencing the effects of those thoughts. But the good news is in every moment you can re-choose the reality you would like to experience.

The teachings of Abraham Hicks explain that maintaining a single thought for only 17 seconds brings a creation well on its way into our experience. The problem with most of us is that we can't seem to keep focused on one thing for very long. Just try meditating on your breath for even a few minutes and watch all the stray thoughts that try and intrude on your silence. What's even worse than being unable to focus on a single thought for any length of time, is that we keep changing our mind. When we keep changing our mind, we're making it harder for the Universe to deliver. We are asking the forces of the Universe to literally keep changing direction. But if we keep focused on what we want with all the intensity of our being, we make it much easier for the Universe to deliver that which we desire. Try and become very clear about what you want and what it would be like for you to have it. Ask yourself, "How would I feel?" "What would it look like?" "What would I do with it?" "How would I most enjoy it?"

If you find you're having difficulty getting clear about your goals, wants and desires, here are some set ups and reminders you might try:

KC   Even though I don't know what I really want, I'm open to the possibility of becoming clear about it.

KC   Even though I can't seem to make decisions about what I want, I'm open to the possibility of realizing what I truly desire.

KC   Even though I can't seem to get clear about what I really want, I'm open to the possibility of my dreams coming true.

EB	I don't know what I want
SE	I've never been able to have what I want
UE	So I've never had to decide what I want
UN	So now I don't know how I feel about things
CH	I'm not certain what I truly want
CB	I'm confused about what I really want
UA	I don't feel like it could really come true
TH	Maybe I'm not meant to have what I want

EB	I'm willing to be open to knowing what I want
SE	I choose to become more aware of what I want
UE	I know that I've received things I've really wanted before
UN	I know of other people who have realized their dreams
CH	So I know it's possible for me too
CB	I choose to believe in a loving supportive Universe
UA	I choose to realize that everyone deserves abundance
TH	I choose to believe that everyone deserves to be loved and happy, even me

So now that you've tapped for your barriers to knowing what you really want, ask yourself, "Who do I want to be, and what do I want to do or have in my life?" Anything is possible. I've included some excellent exercises at the end of this chapter designed to help you flex your muscles of desire (not those muscles!) and begin focusing on what would truly make your heart sing.

Barriers to Abundance

If we're not experiencing true abundance in our lives, it's most likely because we're harboring some unconscious beliefs which prevent us from accepting it into our lives. But in order to receive the abundance that's waiting for us, we must first believe we deserve it, and second, believe that it's possible for us to have it. Because as Abraham Hicks so wisely put it, "The Universe holds within it the ability to manifest any desire you may hold." So the only thing standing between us and our fondest desires is our own lack of belief. If you're not currently experiencing abundance, you may want to take a closer look at your beliefs about money and prosperity.

For example, do you believe that money is the root of all evil? Do you believe that money is not "spiritual"? What do you think about rich people? Do you think it's somehow virtuous to be poor? What did your parents and teachers have to say on the subject of money as you were growing up? List your thoughts about money and wealth here:

_____

_____

_____

_____

_____

_____

If you grew up in a religious tradition that considered money "evil" or looked down on people who had money, those beliefs and ideas are probably still with you today affecting your current level of prosperity. For instance, we may associate poverty with being spiritual or being "Christian". But if we were to take a closer look at the example of Jesus, we see that nothing could be further from the truth. Jesus was a teacher of abundance. In John 10:10 he says, "I came that they would have life, and have it to the full." He also famously multiplied the loaves and the fishes, until there was more than enough for all the hungry people. So much so, that the remainders had to be collected in 12 baskets.

At the wedding in Cana, he transformed water into the choicest of wine. In fact, Christ was so trusting in the abundant goodness of the Universe, in Luke 22:35 it says: 'Then Jesus asked them, "When I sent you without purse, bag or sandals, did you lack anything?" "Nothing," they answered.' This shows us Christ's complete faith in the abundant goodness of a loving Father. In fact, there is nothing inherently noble about being poor. Poverty is really just our demonstration that we don't have faith that we can receive God's bounty for ourselves. It is also wise to consider that the less we have, the less we have to give to others. Whereas the more abundance we have, the more we are able to share with the world.

So let's do some tapping right now for any barriers we might have to receiving full abundance into our lives. First tap on your thoughts about money that you wrote out on the previous page. Then when you're finished, here are some set ups that you might also find helpful:

KC   Even though I don't feel wealthy or abundant right now, I deeply and completely love and accept myself.

KC   Even though I'm afraid I'll never be wealthy, I deeply and profoundly love and accept myself anyway.

KC   Even though I don't believe that I can have what I want, I deeply and completely love and accept myself anyway.

EB   Even though I don't feel abundant in my life right now
SE   I don't have enough in my life
UE   I seem to be conflicted about wealth and abundance
UN   Because other people always seem to have more than I do

CH	Other people are rich and I'm not, it's just not fair
CB	All I seem to have is scarcity and lack
UA	I have all these debts and bills
TH	As soon as I get any money at all, another bill comes in the mail

EB	I feel like a part of me doesn't think I deserve abundance
SE	A part of me doesn't feel worthy of success
UE	A part of me doesn't believe I deserve it
UN	I'm afraid to believe I can have what I want
CH	I must not believe I deserve to have good things happen to me
CB	I must have a block to receiving money and abundance
UA	I don't want to get my hopes up only to have my dreams dashed
TH	I don't want to be disappointed yet again

KC Even though a part of me believes it's wrong to want money, I deeply and completely love and accept myself.

KC Even though money is the root of all evil, I deeply and profoundly love and accept myself anyway.

KC Even though a part of me doesn't believe that God wants me to have money, I choose to recognize that God has only love for me and wants me to be happy.

EB   Even though I think money isn't spiritual

SE   Even though money is the root of all evil

UE   And I think it's wrong for me to be wealthy when others are poor and starving

UN   Even though a part of me believes rich people are greedy

CH   And I just want to be a good person

CB   I choose to see that the more I have, the more I can give to others and help the world

UA   I choose to believe that everyone is worthy of abundance, including me

TH   I choose to understand that God/Spirit/the Universe/Love wants me to be happy, abundant and prosperous

KC   Even though all I can think of is how money brings problems with it, I deeply and completely love and accept myself.

KC   Even though I don't know how I would handle being rich, I deeply and profoundly love and accept myself.

KC   Even though I don't know the first thing about being wealthy, I choose to deeply and completely love and accept myself anyway.

EB   Even though I don't know how to become wealthy

SE   And I'd probably have to work too hard to earn lots of money

UE   And I don't want to work that hard

UN   Even though I don't know how to be rich

CH   And I'm probably not smart enough

CB   I'm willing to see that being abundant is effortless

UA   I'm willing to choose to believe in my ability to manifest my dreams

TH   I choose to believe in my own power to manifest my desires

EB   Even though if I had a lot of money the IRS would probably just take it anyway

SE   I'd probably end up with more bills too

UE   My family might resent me for being rich

UN   My friends might resent me for being wealthy

CH   Even though people would only like me for my money

UA   I am willing to see it differently

TH   I am willing to choose to accept wealth and abundance into my life now

EB   I choose to appreciate all the good things I have right now

SE   I choose to realize that I actually have a lot of prosperity right now

UE   I can begin being grateful for all the good things in my life right now

UN   I choose to feel grateful for my good friends

CH   I choose to feel the abundance that I have at this moment

CB   I choose to see all the abundance that exists in the world around me

UA   I love knowing that even greater abundance is coming to me now

TH   I choose to experience more joy, abundance and wealth every day

Now that you've had a chance to work through your issues surrounding abundance, here are some exercises designed to hone your manifesting skills. They don't necessarily need to be done in order, just start with the one that resonates with you the most.

🦋 Exercise: Vision Board

One exercise that I do faithfully every year on New Year's Eve (although it can be done at any time) is a Vision Board. I get together with a few of my closest friends and they each bring a stack of magazines and a foam core poster board. We listen to music, have refreshments and chat while waiting for the New Years ball to drop in Times Square. All the while, we cut out pictures, words and phrases from the magazines that embody everything we want to experience in our lives during the coming year. We then glue them onto the poster board, creating a beautiful piece of artwork that inspires us and makes us feel joyful. Each time we look at our board, we're excited, knowing that the experiences of our desires are on their way to us even at that very moment.

Something I really enjoy about my boards is looking at the pictures and words on them and seeing how many of them have come to fruition. On one of my boards, I had put the words "I lost 50 pounds" which I had cut out of a fashion magazine. I was very excited to realize that it had come true the very year I had put it on my board. On another I had put the word "passion" in the hopes that I would discover a meaningful and exciting career. That was the year that ThinStead was born. I encourage everyone to make a vision board at least once a year, if not more often. It's a very creative process that helps you identify what your dreams are, and lets you enjoy the process of manifesting them.

Here's what you'll need to make your own vision board:

A piece of white, foam core poster board
Your favorite magazines
Scissors
A Glue Stick
Any decorative items you may want (glitter, puffy paint, ribbons, etc.)

In preparation for making your vision board, think about all the things you'd love to see enter your life. It could be something as grand and abstract as "fulfillment" or as small and simply joyful as a shiny new toaster. Nothing is off limits. It's your life, and they are your dreams. You can select things like money, abundance, a new home or car, vacations, relationships, pets, health, exercise, spirituality, a new career – anything. I also discovered quite by accident, that as a woman I'm very verbal, and I respond especially well to words and phrases on my vision board. I found that putting meaningful phrases on my board elicited a sense of excitement within me, and was very effective for manifesting those conditions within my life. I like to use words like love, passion, freedom, peace, fulfillment, abundance, travel, success, etc. The bottom line is to make your board pleasing to you. It should inspire a sense of excitement, possibility and wonder whenever you look at it. The sky's the limit!

🦋 Exercise: List of Your Wildest Dreams

Another exercise that I highly recommend is to make a list of your wildest dreams and desires. Simply take out a few sheets of paper and at the top write My Wildest Dreams, and then number from 1 to 100 down the left hand margin of the paper. Then after each number, draw a line on which to write one of your wildest dreams. About 25 to 30 lines per page should give you enough room.

Now list as many of your dreams, goals and desires as you can possibly think of. At first it may be hard to come up with 100. But really try to list as many as you can think of. Over time, you might think of other things to add to your list. For example, you might be doing the dishes one morning and you look out the window and you realize, "Gee, I'd really like a new umbrella for the patio table..." Write it down on your list!

Now the object of this list is not to write down what you think you should want, or what anyone else thinks you should want. Also, for the purposes of this list you're not allowed to limit yourself because you think something can't happen, or because you don't know how you can afford it, or how it will come about. This is not the "List of Reasonable Goals". This is the "List of Your Wildest Dreams". Do your best to make them wild! Notice how good imagining all those wonderful experiences and fun stuff feels if you don't tell yourself you can't have them. Anything is acceptable to put on your list as long as you would really and truly like it to happen. There is no judgment here about whether something is a "worthy" goal or not. The only rule is that it be something you truly desire. It can be an experience, a feeling, a relationship, a person, a quality, or a thing. It can be something as big as winning the lottery, or something as small as a great haircut. You decide!

Your list may look something like this:

1.   A brand new car

2.   Weigh 120 pounds

3.   Pay off my credit cards

5.   To know what I want to do with my life

6.   Find a tennis class close by

7.   A new king size bed

8.   Inner peace

9.   A garden full of poppies

10.   A trip to Italy

You get the idea. No desire is too big or too small for your list. To help you zero in on your deepest desires, ask yourself the following questions:

If you could be, do or have anything in your life, and you knew you couldn't fail, what would it be?

_____

_____

_____

_____

_____

Imagine you received 100 million dollars in lottery winnings in your bank account yesterday. What would you do with it?

_____

_____

_____

_____

_____

Who would you become?

_____

_____

_____

_____

_____

Where would you go?

_____

_____

_____

_____

_____

What would you buy?

_____

_____

_____

_____

_____

What would you add to your life?

_____

_____

_____

_____

What would you choose to let go?

_____

_____

_____

_____

Now begin making your list of your wildest dreams!

Getting An Attitude Adjustment

It's been said that the key to the law of attraction is remaining in a positive vibration. The problem is that most of us are trained from birth to focus on the negative or what we don't want in our lives. The trick is then to shift our focus from that which we'd rather not have in our lives to what is currently working. That means focusing on our health, relationships, gifts or abilities, or any other thing which currently provides us with immense satisfaction. There are a number of practices we can engage in which can help shift our focus and nurture a sense of positivity within us. Here are a few exercises that can help:

🦋 Exercise: The Gratitude Attitude

Think about an area of your life that is working well or provides you with great sense of satisfaction. This could be a friendship or other relationship, the beauty of nature, a hobby, an enjoyable activity or a beloved pet.

While remaining focused on this person or thing, write as many pages as you can describing how they/it provides you will comfort, pleasure and enjoyment. While you're writing, feel the abundance you receive from having this person or thing in your life. Write as much and for as long as you can, extolling the virtues of this positive influence in your life. If there are other areas of your life that are bringing you pleasure, write about those too. You can do this practice before you go to bed at night or in the morning when you wake up to set the tone for the day. You can do it whenever you experience some upset during the day, or when you feel yourself dwelling on the negative. Some of my clients have made writing in their gratitude journal a daily practice because they find it so uplifting.

🦋 Exercise: Bless Your Path

You've probably heard that it is more blessed to give than receive. But what does it mean to be "blessed"? Well, a blessing means to receive something good, of course. So what that old familiar axiom means is that giving actually blesses us with receiving greater good. Because like attracts like. This "good" can take the form of prosperity, good feelings and wishes from others, greater opportunities, inner peace or happiness.

But what happens when you don't feel like you have anything to give? Even though you may be temporarily short on cash, you still always have something to give. You could give your time, your talents, a smile, or even a blessing. You can always send your good intentions for others as a blessing to them. Try this blessing exercise for one day, and I think you'll be hooked. You'll begin to feel so good and blessed, you probably won't want to stop.

The way it works is to feel and mentally say "Bless you", or "God bless you" or "May you be blessed" to every person or object you come into contact with. When you say it, try and feel the genuine emotion of wishing the best for another. This can be a real challenge when we encounter someone who is difficult or that we actively dislike. But every person, no matter how difficult, is still a spiritual being on their own perfect path, and they're progressing exactly as they need to. Your blessing for their highest good can be a help on their path to their spiritual evolution. Your act of blessing does a double service, it is a help to the other person and a benefit to your own spiritual growth as well.

It may feel a little funny at first to bless an inanimate object, but in reality all things are alive with spiritual energy. People and objects are all made up of molecules, made up of atoms, made up of subatomic particles, and ultimately space filled with energy. Everything in the Universe is made up of the exact same primal substance. Remember that your simple act of blessing another always comes back to bless you as well.

It's my hope that you found the exercises in this chapter both helpful and uplifting. They can be done any time, and they can be done as often as you like. They're great tools for helping you become more positive in your outlook and start creating a more exciting and fulfilling life.

Chapter 12

Forging A New Life – Addiction Free

As you may have realized by now, ThinStead isn't just about permanent weight loss and freedom from food addiction. It's also about improving your life for the better. The real magic of the program is its ability to give people their hopes, dreams, desires and passion back. The ThinStead program is designed to be a powerful tool for eliminating negative emotions and limiting beliefs and it is one that we can continue to use throughout our lives. Any time we feel angry, sad, guilty or embarrassed, we can take a moment to tap away those feelings. EFT can enhance every area of our lives. Over time, as you use EFT, you will start to become happier and more confident. Your relationships will improve because you're less reactive. Your quality of life will improve immeasurably.

Occasionally a client will come to me and say they didn't feel anything after tapping. That's usually a clear signal to me that they haven't been able to get in touch with the emotions that are causing their addiction yet. Because it's been my experience that if the correct emotional aspects have been identified and released, their food addiction will resolve itself. If you feel you might be encountering some kind of blockage in dealing with your compulsive eating, here are a few things I recommend:

1.   Pay attention to your dreams.

Dreams are very symbolic and often contain strong emotional themes. If you happen to awaken from a dream and feel sadness or anger, tap for that emotion and for the events which took place in your dream. You may find, as my client Karen did, that your dreams could contain the key to overcoming your problems with food.

2.   Tap whenever you feel a strong emotion.

If you're not making significant progress in your healing, it's probably because you've been out of touch with your emotions for a very long time. I recommend tapping immediately whenever you DO happen to experience a strong negative emotion. Whether you happen to be watching a sad movie or TV show, or having an argument with someone, take the time to stop and tap on your feelings of sadness, anger, betrayal, or sense of life being unfair. These emotions are very much tied into your food addiction, and they can act as a doorway to your healing.

3.   Consult a professional.

As I mentioned earlier, working with another person can often help you gain insights into your emotions, motivations and behaviors that you may not have been able to access on your own. Working with a food addiction counselor or qualified therapist can often be a very strong catalyst for change and might be just the push needed to move you forward. Many therapists these days also use EFT to augment and increase the effectiveness of their therapeutic practice, and are quite skilled in helping clients get to the root of their problems.

I've been using EFT for close to a decade now in my own life, and I know firsthand how truly effective it is. The key to success is to keep digging until we reach the specific emotions which are at the core of our food addiction problems. I've used EFT for the emotional pain I've experienced in my past, as well as for minor upsets that crop up from time to time in everyday living. Now and again I'll also receive brief insights into my feelings, behavior patterns and beliefs which are less than constructive toward my happiness and success, and I tap on those too. The person I am today is vastly different than the person I was as a young adult in my 20's. It's been a remarkable journey and I remain in awe of what I perceive to be one of the greatest tools for healing on the planet - EFT.

I also encourage you to continue your own healing journey, by paying attention to your thoughts and feelings and examining what message they might have for you. Spiritual unfoldment and mental health are a continually evolving process. And the process never ends. Our lives can always be made better by releasing that which is negative, or does not serve us. Happiness, peace and tranquility **are** possible. We just have to be willing to release our pain and embrace gentleness, by treating ourselves with kindness, self-love and understanding. Continue using EFT for your daily upsets, spontaneous insights or relationship issues, and watch how your life changes for the better every day.

I'm sure there are many people in your life who could also benefit from the wisdom contained in this book. Why not share the message of ThinStead with your friends and family members? Their lives will be transformed, and they will have you to thank for it.

I also invite you to write to me and share stories of your personal experiences with the ThinStead program. I love to hear each and every one of your moving and powerful stories of personal transformation. It has always been my heart's desire and spiritual goal to help change people's lives for the better, and I'm proud to share ThinStead with you.

I wish you freedom, love and passion on your life's journey!

Kathleen Lammens
www.ThinStead.com

Your life may not have turned out exactly like you planned, but there's still time for it to turn out better than you hoped~

www.ingramcontent.com/pod-product-compliance
Lightning Source LLC
Chambersburg PA
CBHW060837280326
41934CB00007B/814